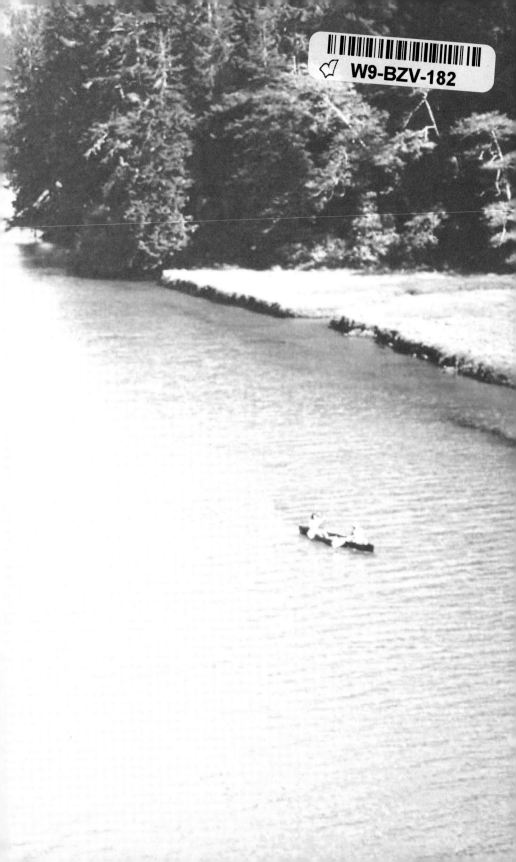

Words of Praise for *Help Me to Heal*

"Bernie Siegel seems to have a knack for lifting patients out of the realm of despondent passivity to an attitude of active anticipation of healing. He hasn't lost his touch. This book can not only change your focus to healing, but can lift you to the high road of a healing environment."

— **C. Everett Koop, M.D., Sc.D.,**
former Surgeon General of the United States

"If you or a loved one have to go through major medical care, the information in this book can be both life-saving and soul-saving. Read it. Absorb it. Use it. These are words of practical, essential wisdom from people who care about you as patients and as human beings."

— **Andrew Weil, M.D.,** Director,
Program in Integrative Medicine, University of Arizona

"Hospital care is currently one of the leading causes of death in the United States. Unfortunately, most of us will require it sooner or later. To help you survive and learn from this experience, and to heal afterwards, Dr. Bernard Siegel and Yosaif August's **Help Me to Heal** *is an invaluable resource."*

— **Larry Dossey, M.D.,**
author of *Healing Beyond the Body;*
Reinventing Medicine; and *Healing Words;*
executive editor, *Alternative Therapies in Health and Medicine*

ॐ

Help Me to Heal

ALSO BY BERNIE SIEGEL, M.D.

Books

Love, Medicine & Miracles (1986)
Peace, Love & Healing (1989)
How to Live Between Office Visits (1993)
Prescriptions for Living (1998)

Audio Books

Love, Medicine & Miracles (two-tape set)
Peace, Love & Healing (two-tape set)
How to Live Between Office Visits (two-tape set)
Prescriptions for Living (two-tape set)

Lectures

How to Never Grow Old and Die Young at Heart
Humor & Healing: Insights on the Positive Effects of Humor for Healing
Insights for Living Well
How to Be an Exceptional Patient

Meditation Audios

Getting Ready: *Meditations for Surgery,*
Chemotherapy, and Other Treatments
Guided Imagery & Meditation
Healing Meditations
Healing Relationships: Your Relationship to Life & Creation

Meditations for Difficult Times: How to Survive & Thrive
Meditations for Enhancing Your Immune System
Meditations for Everyday Living
Meditations for Finding the Key to Good Health
Meditations for Healing Your Inner Child
Meditations for Morning & Evening
Meditations for Overcoming Life's Stresses & Strains
Meditations for Peace of Mind

Affirmation Audios

*Healing Images: Affirmations for Envisioning Yourself
As a Unique Individual*

Video

Affirmations for Living Beyond Cancer
Fight for Your Life
Love, Medicine & Miracles
Healing Spirit
Innervision: Visualizing Super Health
How to Be Exceptional
How to Live Between Office Visits

Please visit the Hay House USA Website at: **www.hayhouse.com;**
the Hay House Australia Website at: **www.hayhouse.com.au;** or the
Hay House U.K. Website at: **www.hayhouse.co.uk**

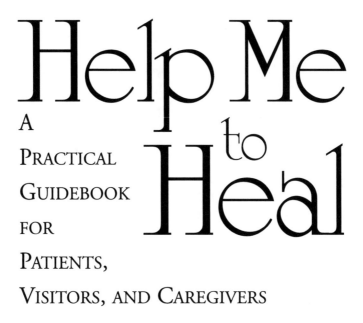

Help Me to Heal

A Practical Guidebook for Patients, Visitors, and Caregivers

Bernie Siegel, M.D., and Yosaif August

HAY HOUSE

Hay House, Inc.
Carlsbad, California • Sydney, Australia • London, U.K.
Canada • Hong Kong

Published and distributed in the United States by: Hay House, Inc., P.O. Box 5100, Carlsbad, CA 92018-5100 • *Phone:* (760) 431-7695 or (800) 654-5126 • *Fax:* (760) 431-6948 or (800) 650-5115 • www.hayhouse.com • **Published and distributed in Australia by:** Hay House Australia Ltd., 18/36 Ralph St., Alexandria NSW 2015 • *Phone:* 612-9669-4299 • *Fax:* 612-9669-4144 • www.hayhouse.com.au • **Published and Distributed in the United Kingdom by:** Hay House UK, Ltd. • Unit 202, Canalot Studios • 222 Kensal Rd., London W10 5BN • *Phone:* 44-20-8962-1230 • *Fax:* 44-20-8962-1239 • www.hayhouse.co.uk • **Distributed in Canada by:** Raincoast • 9050 Shaughnessy St., Vancouver, B.C. V6P 6E5 • *Phone:* (604) 323-7100 • *Fax:* (604) 323-2600

Editorial supervision: Jill Kramer   *Design:* Tricia Proctor

Library of Congress Cataloging-in-Publication Data

Siegel, Bernie S.
 Help me to heal : a practical guidebook for patients, visitors, and caregivers : essential
   tools, strategies and resources for healthy hospitalizations and home convalescence / Bernie S. Siegel and Yosaif August.
 p. cm.
 ISBN 1-4019-0037-2 (Hardcover) — ISBN 1-4019-0060-7 (Tradepaper) 1. Hospital
   patients—Care. 2. Healing. 3. Convalescence. 4. Self-care, Health. 5. Caregivers.
   6. Alternative medicine. I. August, Yosaif. II. Title.
     RA965.6.S56 2003
     362.1'1—dc21
 2003002500   632 0127

                    Hardcover ISBN 1-4019-0037-2
                    Tradepaper ISBN 1-4019-0060-7

                   06 05 04 03   4 3 2 1
                     1st printing, August 2003

To my beloved Bobbie and our children—Jonathan,
   Jeffrey, Stephen, Carolyn, and Keith;
To all the exceptional patients who have been my
   teachers;
To our grandchildren Charles, Samuel, Gabriel,
   Elijah, Simone, Jarrod, Patrick, and Jason;
And to all the grand children of the world:
May you all feel loved enough to heal the world,
And in your lifetime see the end of man's inhumanity
   to man.

— **Bernie Siegel, M.D.**

ॐ

To Tsurah, my love, co-journeyer, and joyful
   dance partner;
To Max and Anne August and Jean London, teachers
   about life, love, happiness, and healing;
To Irwin Kritchek, who taught us what being there
   for each other truly means;
To Marika, Luke, and Gail; and to Harry, Raphael,
   and all the beautiful children who take our
   breath away!

— **Yosaif August**

CONTENTS

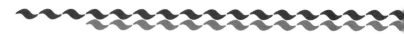

Preface xiii
Acknowledgments xvii
Introduction: Why You Need to Be Empowered .xix

PART I: A PATIENT'S SURVIVAL GUIDE
Chapter 1:   Empowering Yourself and Your Team 3
Chapter 2:   Healing and How It Happens 17
Chapter 3:   Preparing for a Healthy Hospitalization 35
Chapter 4:   Crossing the Threshold: How to Behave Like a Respant
              in the Hospital 59
Chapter 5:   Creating Vital Signs 79
Chapter 6:   Healing Encounters: Tips on Creating Visits That
              Help You to Heal 87
Chapter 7:   Prescriptions for Self-Healing .97
Chapter 8:   Getting Out: Continuing the Process of Healing 105
Chapter 9:   Healing at Home: Staying Empowered 115

**PART II: HEALING STRATEGIES FOR FAMILY,
FRIENDS, AND CAREGIVERS**
Chapter 10:   Being an Empowering Advocate 129
Chapter 11:   How to Be a Healing Visitor .145
Chapter 12:   Healing for the Caregiver 159

PART III: HEALING WAYS
Chapter 13:   Activities That Heal 171
           • Tips for Patients: Turning Bedside Visits into
             Healing Encounters
           • Tips for Families, Bedside Companions, and Visitors
           • Bedside Yoga
           • Walking and Wheelchairing
           • Massage: The Healing Power of Touch
           • Bernie's Resource List
           • Yosaif's Resource List
           • Entitlement Learner's Permit

Afterword: Passwords 191
Self-Help Resources 193
About the Authors 211

Help Me to Heal

Lord, help me to heal.
Restore me to health;
Bring harmony into my life,
And into my body.

Lord, help me to heal.
Fill my soul with a
Longing for life;
Give me the vision to
See my own perfection.

Lord, help me to heal.
To cleanse my mind of
All doubt and despair;
To rise above the illusion
Of time and disease.

Lord, help me to heal.
To know only love,
And feel only love
In the purity of my heart.

Lord, help me to heal.
Make me stronger in faith;
By your grace bring me to
Peace of mind.

Lord, help me to heal.
Let me know the bounty
Of your love and power;
Restore me to wholeness.

Lord, help me to heal.
Show me how to surrender
Completely to your will;
Lift me into your arms
And hold me like
A newborn babe.

Help me to smile again
With all my heart and soul.

— **Bob Silverstein**, 3/31/98
(Used by permission of the author)

PREFACE

Yosaif and I met, for the first time, at a conference where I was a keynote speaker and he was presenting a workshop on "Nurturing the Caregiver." After the conference, we started a lively and playful e-mail relationship and discovered that we had similar perspectives on healing. Early on, Yosaif sent me a sample Bedscape® (a window-sized photomural that can be hung on hospital curtains, providing patients with a more relaxing healing environment). I liked it and started telling people in health care about it.

Next, he sent me an early version of this book, then called *Creative Visiting,* and asked me to write an Introduction. I was impressed with the project but didn't have time to contribute to it, so I offered to write an endorsement instead. That was the last I heard of the book until several years later, when Yosaif asked me to join him as co-author and help expand the scope of the book.

Again, I thought it was a great idea, but I was still too busy. However, one night after I received Yosaif's second invitation, I came across some writing I'd done advising patients to pack themselves a "Siegel Kit," complete with mischievous props such as water pistols and Magic Markers. It struck me that the Siegel Kit fit perfectly with the book Yosaif was contemplating, so I e-mailed him that very night, saying "I think God is telling me to do this project with you."

We agreed to collaborate on a book, which we decided to call *Patient No More.* We chose that title to emphasize the importance of being empowered and paying attention to *all* of your needs—physical, mental, and spiritual. Our main concern was to ensure that your medical care didn't focus solely on your biology while ignoring your humanity and healing—we wanted you to be cared for as an individual rather than treated as a disease. In *Patient No More,* we hoped to coach you in empowerment, self-knowledge, and the expression of your inner being.

Soon after we started, however, we found ourselves writing about much more than what we'd set out to, and the title *Patient No More* began to seem too adversarial and limited. We wanted you to be empowered, but we also wanted you to know that there are many ways you can help yourself heal, whether you're in the hospital or convalescing at home.

We knew that the information people needed to organize their own healing process isn't usually given to patients and their families, and surprisingly, most medical professionals don't get this information in their training either, although it's not new. People have known for decades that the mind and body communicate. Seventy years ago, Carl Jung was presented with a patient's dream about a blockage in a pond of milky fluid. Jung analyzed the dream and concluded that the man had a brain tumor blocking the flow of his cerebrospinal fluid. Jung's diagnosis was correct, but how many medical students today are being taught that dream analysis can be a useful medical resource?

We wrote this book to give you the tools you'll need to make decisions that are right for you and that'll get you the attention and care you require, whether in a hospital, nursing home, doctor's office, rehabilitation center, or at home. The stories, ideas, and activities in these pages will help you tap in to your own natural healing powers. They'll show you how to supplement your powers with the sources of healing energy around you: your family, friends, neighbors, congregants, health-care professionals, and spiritual connections in whatever form you may experience them.

This book takes a holistic approach in that it encourages you to use all of your resources. Everything we've written is based on three simple assumptions:

1. You are entitled to be healed no matter what your life experience has been.
2. You can learn to create a healing team composed of the significant people in your life.
3. You can learn to become the master of your life's time.

If these assumptions strike you as true and inspiring, you'll find the information in here useful as you set about healing. If you're skeptical about these assumptions, if you doubt that you're entitled to loving care and attention, or if you fear that you'll fail or you don't deserve to be healed, then it's even more important that you consider the wisdom presented here. Before you give up and say that you can't take charge of your own life and healing, why not try some of the techniques for creating a sacred healing space and forming a healing team? Why not combine your inspiration with our information?

You can learn to be open, use new healing approaches, and receive the love and care you deserve. To help you, we've provided an "Entitlement Learner's Permit" in Part III of this book. This permit gives you the right to love and be loved, and to care and be cared for. It's valid until you've learned that you're permanently entitled to loving care. Operating with your learner's permit, you can try some new approaches for turning your doubt and anger into energy that creates change and brings order into your life, even when you're ill and can't control everything that's happening to you.

— **Bernie Siegel, M.D.**

ACKNOWLEDGMENTS

I acknowledge the assistance and dedication of Victoria Pryor, George Liles, Yosaif August, and the editors at Hay House.

— **Bernie Siegel, M.D.**

❅

So many angels!

My beloved Tsurah co-created this vision and has totally supported me all along the way.

Bernie has been an angel from the first time I was personally introduced to him by Joy Hopkins-Hausman.

Gene Schwartz has steadfastly given love, wisdom, inspiration, and more.

My agent and friend, Bob Silverstein of Quicksilver Books, offered us the current title, his prayer/poem that it's based on, and much more.

Victoria Pryor gifted us with her wisdom and experience for orchestrating and midwifing this collaboration.

George Liles brought Bernie's voice and mine together in a very special way.

Jill Kramer, editorial director at Hay House, has extended a strong commitment to this project, and Gwendolyn Tapper generously contributed her intelligence and grace to every aspect of it.

I'm deeply grateful for the wisdom of Ellen Weaver (Bedside Ballet), Stephanie Kristal (Bedside Yoga), Ellie Kramer (physical therapy), and Bruce Isa Franck (massage); to the holistic nurses for sharing their wisdom; and Orrin "Big O" Judd, for encouraging me to resurrect this project.

I'm also grateful to my mentors: Reb Zalman Schachter-Shalomi; Wayne Ruga; Barbara Sarah; Mack Lipkin, M.D.; John Stoeckle, M.D.; Steven Horowitz, M.D.; and Roger Ulrich, Ph.D. Thanks also to Laurance S. Rockefeller; Richard Rockefeller, M.D.; Luke Brussel; Marika Brussel; David Tapper; Deborah Moskowitz; Tory Ettlinger; Harris Breiman; Rob Cohen; Ravi Ramaswami, M.D.; Veda Andrus; Marie Shanahan; Rabbi Dayle Friedman; Eileen Zenker; Vivien Ubell; Barry Samuels; Kevin Smith; Larry Bush; Meyer Rothberg; Al and Trudy Walker; Roe DiBona; Marvin Beck; Gail Tuchman; Heidi Washburn; Linda Caigan; Linda Zelizer; Steve Abrams; Debra Matza; Sara Marberry; Dena Crane; Arline Cohen; Robert Selkowitz; Dan Gottesman; Jill Hall; Kay Trimmer; Shlomo Cooperstein; Paul Brenner; Jeanne Anselmo; Barbara and Larry Dossey; Herschel Kranitz; Jain Malkin; Michael McGarvey, M.D.; Thomas DelBanco, M.D.; Lorayne Mion; Mardelle Shepley; Bill and Judy Thomas; Mark Lewis; Joe McBride; Jane Tollett; Mary Elizabeth Boyd; Coy Smith; Franne Entelis; Carol Jones; Noah Klarish; Michael Lean; Jule Malowitz; Ruth McCaffrey; Tamara Horton; Ruth Vanden Bosch; and Leben and Gezunzein.

Special thanks to the many others who offered ideas and healing stories we weren't able to include in this edition of *Help Me to Heal.*

Last, not least, are Feivel "The Raifeh" (my great-grandfather), and Francine "One in Nine" Kritchek, for showing how to turn life's personal challenges into healing for others.

— **Yosaif August**

꒰꒱

INTRODUCTION

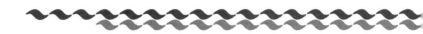

Why You Need to Be Empowered

In recent years, we've been bombarded with stories about how dangerous it is to be hospitalized. While we were writing this Introduction, an issue of *Prevention* magazine featured a cover story entitled "Get Out of the Hospital Alive." At the same time, newspapers were reporting that a little girl who went into the operating room to have her tonsils removed had eye surgery instead, while the child who needed eye surgery had a tonsillectomy. In a major teaching hospital, two people recently died during cardiac catheterizations because the oxygen and nitrous oxide lines were reversed, and people across the world mourned the death of Jesica Santillan—the 17-year-old girl who died after doctors performed a heart-and-lung transplant using organs of the wrong blood type.

The news is full of horror stories about the wrong organs being removed and the wrong limbs being amputated. But the scariest part of the story is that medical mistakes happen every day. Just look at the statistics: In the United States, hospitalization is one of the ten leading causes of death, with ten people per hour dying in these institutions because of medical mistakes. Maybe what we really need is a book called *Help Me to <u>Survive</u>*.

If you think that the situation couldn't possibly be that bad, be aware that the Institute of Medicine (IOM) has estimated that as many as 98,000 people die each year due to medical blunders. In response to the IOM's 1999 report, the Joint Commission on Accreditation of Healthcare Organizations (JCAHO) has launched a campaign with the message "Speak Up: Help Prevent Errors in Your Care." Their brochure offers the following suggestions on how you can avoid being the victim of medical errors. To obtain a copy of the full brochure, call JCAHO at 877-223-6866, or log on to their Website at **www.jcaho.org**:

- Ask your doctor about the specialized training and experience that qualifies him or her to treat your illness (and be sure to ask the same questions of those physicians to whom he or she refers you). [If your doctor doesn't want to answer questions, find another caregiver.]

- Make sure you can read the handwriting on any prescriptions written by your doctor. If you can't read it, the pharmacist may not be able to either.

- Understand that more tests or medications may not always be better. Ask your doctor what a new test or medication is likely to achieve. [And don't forget that some alternative treatments are more effective and less risky, and are often less costly.]

There are many other questions you can ask to protect yourself from medical errors, and they all hinge on your being empowered so you won't be intimidated when you need to get information.

So how did hospitals get to be such dangerous places? We think it happened when medical technology began to replace care. Technology may save lives, but it can't take the place of the consideration that one person can provide for another. With few exceptions, doctors, nurses, and other health-care providers are taught a lot about technology but little if anything about how to provide personal attention. They don't learn to take into account the patient's experience, or their emotional and spiritual issues.

Hospitals would be run very differently if administrators had to live in the facilities they operate. We sometimes say that the fastest way to improve the quality of care given in hospitals would be to employ only those health-care professionals who have spent at least a week as a patient. When doctors experience serious illness—either their own or a loved one's—they often become advocates for patient empowerment.

One such physician created a survival list after he was hospitalized, and nothing on his list came from his medical-school education. It would be great if insurance companies gave patients a copy of the list, which included such useful tips as, "Write on your knee: 'Cut here.'" What if one set of parents had written "Cut here" on their daughter's forehead, above the eye that needed the operation; and the other parents had written "Remove tonsils and adenoids only" on their daughter's chin? Those children wouldn't have undergone the wrong operations.

The JCAHO offers similar advice, but they go one step further—they urge patients to "mark not only the site that is to be operated on, but also the one that should not be touched." In one hospital, after someone had amputated the wrong leg, the medical staff decided that in the future they'd write "no" on the healthy leg. But when the orderly writes "no" on your leg, does that mean "No, not this one," or does it mean "This leg is no good"? If you want to be safe, make your message clear and unambiguous. One woman about to have breast surgery wrote, "Not this one, stupid." Her message left no room for misunderstanding.

That same physician's survival list ended by advising patients to be assertive, ask questions, and not worry about annoying the hospital staff. He's right. Being a good patient isn't your goal; staying alive is. You want to avoid medical mishaps, so if you sense that something is wrong with your treatment, insist that the staff stop and verify the details. You don't have to make headlines and be involved in lawsuits—you don't need to give anyone permission to take your life.

The word *hospital* is derived from *hospitality,* but medical care today rarely involves the latter. Any hotel manager knows how to make people feel comfortable and safe. Why shouldn't health-care professionals know as much about taking care of people? (Likewise, we notify hotel staff of our needs in advance. Why not do the same with hospitals?)

❧

Psychologists, massage therapists, and advertisers know that colors, textures, sounds, sights, and aromas can contribute to our peace of mind—it's a fact that's been demonstrated in scientific studies. But how many modern cancer centers take the trouble to introduce pleasant sounds and smells? When patients become anxious and restless during an MRI and they can't lie still, the test has to be cancelled; the patient's diagnostic workup is delayed and the hospital loses money. A major cancer center learned that if you play music and fill the room with a soothing aroma, patients relax and money is saved.

Horst Schulze, the former president and COO of The Ritz-Carlton Hotel Company, learned from his experience as a cancer patient how to improve his hotels. He decided that his business should be to make people feel cared for—the way he wished he'd been treated in the hospital. Everyone working at one of the Ritz-Carlton hotels is given a list of "Gold Standards" that instructs them on how to accommodate their guests. It begins like this: "We are ladies and gentleman caring for ladies and gentlemen," and it goes on to say, "The genuine care and comfort of our guests is our highest mission."

By way of comparison, the oath of the American College of Surgeons says: "I promise to deal with each patient as I would wish to be dealt if I were in the patient's position." Would you rather be cared for by ladies and gentlemen, or "dealt with"? We think that when someone is "dealing with" you, or with your diagnosis, they are more likely to perform the wrong operation.

The hotel's principles are better from the staff's point of view, too. "Dealing with" people is much less satisfying than "caring for" them, which may explain why it's hard to find enough nurses to work in hospitals while the Ritz-Carlton staff has only a 5-percent annual turnover rate.

※

This book is for people who are searching for information—people like a young woman with cancer who wrote to us recently. "I was admitted to the hospital the day I was diagnosed," she wrote, "and my frantic parents drove up to be with me." At the hospital, she and her family had the kind of experience we've been describing: The hospital staff wasn't caring for her or listening to her and her family, so she acted like a survivor. She quickly checked out of that hospital and found a new doctor and hospital that *would* provide proper care. She started reading inspirational books, meditating, using guided imagery, and watching healing videos that were available at the new hospital. That young woman is on the path to healing, and she's now thankful for the cancer that changed her life. "My illness has opened up a door of reality that a healthy person can't understand," she wrote. "I know I can't live my life in fear."

We put this book together to provide a resource for people such as that young woman who was diagnosed with cancer. Part I is a survival guide addressed to anyone who is ill, Part II is geared to visitors and caregivers, and Part III contains practical guidance and instructions for healing activities. We hope that people who are ill will also read the pages for visitors and caregivers so that they'll know how to help others help them. Likewise, it's our intention that visitors and caregivers read "A Patient's Survival Guide" (Part I) to learn more about the needs of their loved ones.

If you're like the young woman who changed hospitals the day she was admitted—if you have the courage she has—then we have the information you need. We know from years of experience that the information collected here can help you heal—whether you're hospitalized, convalescing at home, or in an assisted-living facility.

Because it's difficult for disease to exist in a body filled with love, your healing may result in a cure. However, we never promise cures, and we never advise people to do things solely to avoid dying. If we were to guarantee cures, people would get mad at us because eventually they're going to die, and then in heaven they'd need group therapy to learn to forgive us. So please, don't read this book to avoid death. Read it to heal your life, and to receive the blessings that come in many shapes and sizes—one of which may be learning that the treatments and side effects of your disease are not all negative.

If you want to heal, you must be willing to change. No book or person can change you—only you can change yourself. If you have the inspiration, we can guide, coach, and assist you in mobilizing your resources. We can help you develop the will to live and the strength to survive, and we can show you what you need to know in order to say to your family, friends, and treatment team: *"Help me to heal."*

꙳

Authors' Note: *We've prefaced certain blocks of copy throughout the book with our individual names to differentiate between our respective voices.*

— Bernie and Yosaif

PART I

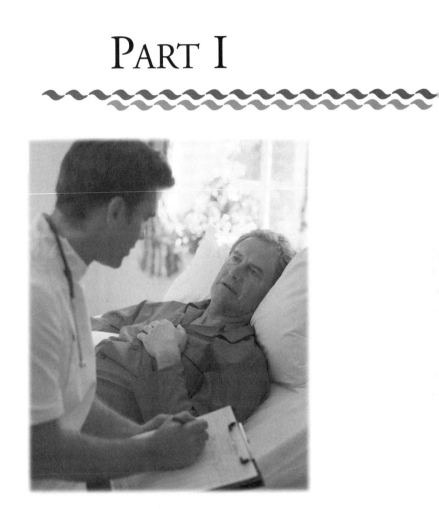

A Patient's
Survival Guide

CHAPTER 1

Empowering Yourself and Your Team

When you know that you're going to spend time in a hospital, you can prepare in advance for a successful stay. If you have a chronic condition that will require long-term care, you may have had plenty of time to gather the information you'll need to make decisions about your treatment—by reading books about healing, interviewing doctors, and enlisting the support of family and friends to form a healing team. If you're hospitalized due to an emergency or traumatic injury, however, you probably didn't have the luxury of preparing yourself for the situation.

But no matter how much or how little you've been able to plan ahead, there's one thing you can do almost immediately to make certain that you receive quality care: *Be empowered.* If you want to heal while you're hospitalized or convalescing in another setting, then you need to take control of your situation. We all face difficulties in life, but those who are empowered know that they can choose how they'll respond. When these people become ill, they make proactive decisions about their care and treatment. They know that as long as they're calling the shots, the disease isn't controlling their lives. They're still in charge, and that's the first step in healing. It may also lead to a cure, because when changes are made in attitude, changes begin to occur in the body as well.

If you're empowered, you'll make noise, move, and display emotions when you're confronted with difficulties; you won't try to be the strong, silent type. You can't afford to internalize your anger and try to please everyone involved in your care—you can make yourself sicker with that kind of behavior. You need to speak out, make your needs known, and express your feelings. If your goal is healing, then you need to ask questions and not worry about how other people will react. It doesn't matter what they think; what matters is getting the information you need to put yourself on the path to inner peace and healing.

Unfortunately, before getting sick, many people don't ever stop to think about who's making the important decisions in their lives. When faced with a serious illness, they begin to evaluate for the first time how they're spending their time and who's really making the key choices for them. This self-assessment can lead to fundamental changes, and many newly empowered people end up being grateful for the illness that finally made them think profoundly about their existence and prevented them from letting others dictate how they'll live. After all, there are blessings in every curse.

While it's always the right time to become empowered, it's especially important to take charge of yourself when you must interact with nurses, doctors, and other medical professionals. Unless your health-care practitioners (or their families) have recently experienced a serious illness and hospitalization, they have no idea what you're going through. They may be very good at treating your biology and diagnosis, but that doesn't mean that they'll pay any attention to your needs as a person. You have to be able to let them know what you're going through if you want them to have some sense of what you need beyond a prescription or procedure.

Most doctors are fascinated by the human body, but few are as interested in the person who comes with that body. If you're empowered, you'll let your physicians know that *you* come with your body, and you'll make decisions about your treatment. It's fine to ask nurses, "Which doctor would you use if you were in my situation?" The nurses know who the caring and capable physicians are, and you need to know, too. You can find out by asking open-ended questions such as, "Which doctors are easy to work with? Which ones listen to the nurses?" You can also learn about doctors by watching their interaction with nurses—is the doctor someone they respect and enjoy working with? Does he or she accept constructive criticism? Generally, any physician who accepts criticism and says, "I'm sorry," is a competent and caring professional.

You also have to continue to ask questions about every aspect of your treatment. If a doctor wants to know why you're inquiring, say, "Because it's my illness, and I have to decide whether to accept the treatment you're prescribing."

We want to show you how to become empowered so that you can get the best possible care. We'll tell you about people who were assertive, healed their lives, and lived longer than their doctors expected. But we need to warn you that reading these stories won't heal you. Healing is not simply a question of accumulating information. If our lessons about healing have any effect, it will be because you've had the desire and determination to *act* on what you've learned.

What Empowered Patients Do

Exactly what will you say or do when you're empowered? Here are some examples from several sources, including a physician who was hospitalized and a patient who wrote to Ann Landers.

- Form a healing team, and be an active member of that team.

- Have someone from your team in constant attendance, especially when you know you're going to be sedated, unconscious, or unable to defend yourself.

- If you have hearing or visual problems or can't speak, be sure that everyone knows about it—even if you have to wear a sign.

- Don't assume anything. Make sure that all your health-care professionals are aware of your history. Be certain that they're in agreement about your care and are able to communicate with one another.

- Tape a sign and photo on your bed or door listing your name, medical conditions, allergies, and room number.

- Ask anything you want to. There are no foolish questions, and you have the right to answers.

- Always request a second opinion about any treatment you're unsure of.

- Decorate your room to personalize it.

- Make sure that the people caring for you wash their hands.

- Move out of any room with a sneezing or coughing roommate.

- Make sure that the medical staff that's caring for you is healthy and not a source of disease.

- Confirm that any equipment used on you is clean and sterilized.

- Tell your doctor about all medications and supplements you're taking, and ask about any possible interactions with newly prescribed drugs or treatments (for example, do they affect bleeding or cause negative side effects when used in combination with other drugs?).

- Know the names of your medications, proper dosages, and the times you're scheduled to receive them. If your pills look different or aren't brought to you at the expected time, question the nurse.

- Understand why you're taking a medication and whether it has any side effects.

- Notify someone immediately if you think you're having any drug reactions, or if you note a change in your condition or in the way you're feeling.

- If you're going to the operating room, write "Cut here" on the appropriate part of your body with a Magic Marker, and write "Don't cut here" on the other side.

- Choose a hospital where the procedure you're having is done frequently.

- Know your blood type.

- Don't eat hospital food if it doesn't smell or taste right, or if it's served at the wrong time or preoperatively.

- Always ask for your test results and insist that they be explained to you in a layperson's language. For instance, ask what the normal range is and how your results compare with that range.

- When you're discharged, make sure that you're informed about the treatment plan to follow.

- If you feel that someone is making a mistake, say something. Trust your instincts. Even if you're wrong, you'll still be alive.

If you feel unable to carry out any of these tasks, assign it to one of your team members. Let them speak up and make noise for you.

How to Be Empowered

When you're empowered, you'll make decisions based on what feels right for you. Notice that we said "what *feels* right." This is important. It's not a matter of what you *think* is best, because when you're ill and making decisions about your care, you have to use your heart wisdom. You'll know what's right for you if you pay attention to your body's needs. If you don't, you'll suffer more than you need to and find it harder to heal.

Pay attention to pain. Whether it's physical or emotional, pain can help you understand your body and its needs. To appreciate your pain, think of your feelings as an appetite. Pain calls attention to your need for something, just as hunger calls attention to your need for food.

To understand what your pain is telling you, think about how you'd describe your feelings to someone else. The metaphors you use can help you understand what's causing the pain.

Bernie: One woman with severe migraine headaches described her pain as a weight, which seemed like a strange description of pain. Her headache was bad enough to require hospitalization, but as we talked it became clear to her that the weight she was talking about was her marriage. Fifteen minutes after she made this discovery, her headache was gone and she no longer needed hospitalization. Another woman told me she had a stabbing pain in her back, while a man said his pain was a burning sensation.

The woman needed to figure out who she thought was stabbing her in the back, and the man needed to examine what was making him angry (burning him up).

Be honest when people ask, "How are you feeling?" If you're depressed, don't hide it for their sake. Masking your depression will use up energy you can't afford to waste. Don't let yourself get angry, ashamed, or despondent about being depressed—that can put you in a downward spiral and weaken your immune system even more. After all, you don't get upset when you're hungry—when you feel hunger, you seek food. Likewise, when you feel depressed, take the time to listen to your feelings and find what you need to do to nourish your life. A depression, like a disease, can be a gift and a blessing if you let it serve as a wake-up call. Remember that you have a choice: You can have a happy and useful depression if you ask yourself, "Why am I feeling this way? What can I learn from it? What do I need to change in my life?"

Keeping a journal will guide you toward healing decisions. A journal in which you record your schedule and appointments won't provide much insight, but a journal of your feelings can be very helpful. If you store your emotions in your journal, then you won't have to keep them bottled up in your body, where they can be destructive. During the day, make notes on your feelings so that you can expand on them later when you have time to write. Give yourself some Sabbath time, or what we call "white-room time," every day. The white room is a place with no stimulation, distraction, or disturbance, clean and clear of the clutter of life. In the white room, you're free to do whatever you want—rest, create, or focus on your healing.

When you make notes about your feelings, don't forget to record the joy and love you experience.

Bernie: In my early journals, I recorded only my pain. My wife changed my awareness one day when I told her that my life was painful and not funny. She reminded me of the many funny things that happen each day that I'd end up telling the family about at dinner. She was right, but until she pointed it out, I never noticed the light moments or put them into my journals.

Taking white-room time is a way of saying yes to yourself and no to what you don't want to spend your lifetime doing. You know you're empowered when you know when to say yes and when to say no. Saying yes to what you truly want sends your body messages that you want to live. This is important because the mind can either be a very powerful survival tool or a very destructive force, depending on how it's used. Your body knows whether you have a conscious and unconscious will to live, and it responds accordingly.

You may not realize it, but whether you choose the path of empowerment depends to a large extent on whether you love yourself and feel worthwhile. How highly you value yourself, in turn, depends on what you've learned from your parents, teachers, and religion. If you describe your parents as unloving, if your teachers made you feel like a failure, and if you believe in a god who punishes you, you have almost a 100-percent chance of experiencing a major illness by midlife. Why? Because you're more likely to be self-destructive, addicted, and interested in seeking the most easily available pleasure, and less likely to be searching for health and self-empowerment. But no one has to stay on a self-destructive or suicidal course. Instead of ending your life, why not put an end to what's killing you? The goal is to save *your* life, not the life others have imposed on you. If you bring forth what's within you, you can save yourself. If you don't, you'll destroy yourself.

There is one more critical component in healing, and that's relationships. Your connections with people and spiritual powers can save your life. Notice that out of people with the same type of cancer, women live longer than men, and married men outlive single men. In fact, married men who smoke as much as single men are less likely to develop lung cancer. It's not sleeping with estrogen and progesterone that provides the men protection; it's relationships that make the difference. We all need meaning, and relationships bring meaning to our lives. To be healthy, we need to contribute love, and serve someone or something. Many studies have shown that people who care for plants, pets, and other living things have longer lives. One cancer patient we know explained why she's still alive: "I can't die, because there's no one in my family willing to take care of my 20 cats after I'm gone."

Your body's chemistry is altered by all of the above. It's all scientific and bio-logical—not path-o-logical.

Healing Is a Team Sport

Your healing has to begin with you, but that doesn't mean it's something you must do alone. You need a team: doctors, nurses, relatives, friends, loved ones, and anyone else who can be of psychological, physical, or technical assistance. All your caregivers need to work together if you're going to beat your illness by healing your life. We (Bernie and Yosaif) can be your coaches, because we're familiar with what it takes to be a winner, but *you* must be the captain of the team—responsible for selecting the plays, assigning the positions you want other team members to fill, and encouraging everyone to participate wholeheartedly.

If you don't like the sports metaphor, try viewing your healing team as an orchestra. You'll need a variety of instruments: Some require physical strength and make sounds that get everyone's attention, while others take a gentle touch and have a more peaceful influence. You choose who's in the orchestra and what instruments they'll play, and you select the music and conduct the musicians to create harmonies and rhythms that make you feel comfortable.

Whether you view your healing ensemble as a team or an orchestra, the important thing is to acknowledge that when it comes to healing, no one person can do everything. You need specialists who can provide the knowledge and skills your healing requires. And remember that all the members of your team have the right to say no when you need them. Be explicit about this: Explain to your team at the beginning that you're all living under the same survival rules. You may be the only one on the team who's ill, but you still don't know who will die first, so you don't want to take advantage of anyone.

Everyone on the team needs to agree to say no to anything they don't want to do. You don't want people taking care of each other out of guilt or a sense of pity—that kind of giving can lead to resentment and even illness because it's not about love. When people care for each other out of love, the gifts they give benefit both parties.

Just as your teammates have the right to say no to your requests, they also have the right to drop off the team. We all have limited time, our own issues to deal with, and our own lives to heal. If someone does choose to leave the team, let him or her go. Your team is a relay team anyway, and the departing member can pass the baton to the next runner. You may need a new member to replace the person who's dropping off, but you don't necessarily have to be the one who lines up the replacement. The person who is leaving or another member of your team can invite someone else to join.

Don't whine about what your needs are—be honest. Give your team a list so they know what you need and when you need it. Be specific about things as simple as when you want a visit. Let your teammates know if you want someone present every day, or if you'd rather that everyone show up on a weekend. Speak up if you want someone to hold your hand during a painful test or treatment, and remind them to take their rings off so that when you squeeze, it won't hurt them so much.

It's vitally important that you and your team listen to each other. We can't communicate our needs if no one's listening. Be clear that you're not asking the team to cure every complaint, you're only asking them to listen so that you can clarify what your next steps will be. Sometimes you may find that someone on your team has a better perspective of the situation than you do. After listening to your treatment plan, for instance, someone may want you to ask for a second opinion. The decision will ultimately be yours, of course, but you need to listen to your teammates before making it.

As captain of the team, you call the plays, and everyone must understand that they are to represent you even when they don't agree with you. Are they free to criticize your decisions? Yes, because their criticism polishes your mirror. Let them know that you're serious about healing, and that you want to know when you're making mistakes. No one on your team will know everything, and no one should act as if he or she does. People will have differences of opinion, but no one is a villain—not you, not your family, and not your health-care providers. If people are doing a bad job of caring for you, it's usually because they weren't taught how to care for people, or they're hindered by their own fear of the situation.

To get the treatment you need, you and your team must be willing to be assertive. Tell your team to speak up and ask for what you need, and for what *they* need as well. You'll be amazed at how rules can be changed when you're assertive. Say, "No, I'm not going in the operating room without my tape recorder," or "I insist on my spouse being at my bedside in the ICU," or "I want to see my dog in the hospital lobby." Disagree with the recommended treatment, or the manner in which the staff is providing it, and watch what happens.

Bernie: One word of team-building advice specifically for women, especially nurses, who have an ill family member: Don't drain yourself. Say no when you need some white-room time for yourself. Be aware that men usually don't handle emotional problems well. Too often they desert their wives and girlfriends in times of crisis. They have a great deal of difficulty sharing feelings and joining a team, which is something women do as a reflex in times of stress. Men are more likely to take a fight-or-flight approach: If they can't fight it or fix it, they take off. So be prepared. You aren't the problem—the problem is their discomfort, or their dis-ease with disease.

To be a fully empowered patient and healing-team member, you need to be able to step outside gender-defined ways of behaving. If you want to heal, it's important that you be a complete human being and be comfortable with behaviors that are generalized as masculine and feminine. Fortunately, this is somewhat easier than it was in the 1950s. Today people don't find it particularly strange when a man admits to being scared or a woman makes John Wayne look like a wimp when she's unhappy with the care she's receiving. Men and women are generally allowed a wider range of emotions and behavior now, and people may not find it odd that you're feisty when you need to be, and open, receptive, and expressive when circumstances call for that kind of response.

Yosaif: Moving beyond the traditional masculine and feminine roles can be a matter of life and death. I'm fortunate to have been with my dad at two critical junctures in his battle with cancer. He'd lived all his life in a traditional masculine role, but at these two moments I witnessed a man freed from the confines and restraints he usually experienced. The first liberating moment was when he made the very courageous decision to undergo a 16-hour, two-team surgery and then face an extended period of recovery and rehabilitation. In making that brave choice, my father was clearly choosing life, even though it would mean long periods of being cared for. The second moment came when he accepted his surgeon's prognosis that the cancer had recurred and was untreatable. This time my dad's choice was equally courageous, and with great grace, he "surrendered" to this situation.

He embraced his imminent death and spent the final three months of his life completing his relationships with people who were important to him.

To make good choices about healing, you need to know what types of therapies and treatments may be available. This book provides information about how to organize a healing team, but you also need information specific to your illness. If you're empowered, you'll be relentless in pursuit of your best options. A lot of good information is now available on the Internet and in libraries. You can learn more about your disease by chatting with people who have the same affliction.

Yosaif: I remember my friend Steve sitting at his computer keyboard, finding out everything he needed to know about his treatment options after he was diagnosed with prostate cancer. Steve is a thoroughly empowered person, and his computer provided access to the information he needed to make good choices for himself. After successful treatment and a subsequent hip operation, Steve was free from cancer and pain. He later said that his only regret was that he hadn't used the same empowered approach when he and his wife were having their kitchen remodeled.

If you're not able to gather information yourself, you can ask someone on your team to take on this assignment. Sometimes it's better to have a team member do the research, because the hunt for information can bring you into contact with people who are comfortable being victims and who distract you from your healing. They may view their illness as a chance to get attention and avoid responsibility. You do not want to avoid responsibility; you want to *take* responsibility for yourself and make the important decisions about your life.

Let your team make calls and handle the legwork. At times, you may ask the medical staff to tell someone other than you about the possible side effects of your treatment. If you don't know the side effects, you can't induce them through the power of suggestion. Your team members can watch for the side effects while you focus on the benefits of the treatment.

When you're making choices about your healing, look to your intuition for guidance. Involve your team members in this, too. Ask them to share their intuitive feelings about what's right for you. Remember that healing works both ways—you can give a team member a physical or emotional hug, too, when he or she is having a bad day. Later, when you're up to it, you can hold a surprise party for your team to thank them for what they did for you.

Don't ever forget that love and healthy laughter are always appropriate. Make sure that your team knows how important humor is to your healing. Tell them you want humorous get-well cards—this is also a favor you're doing them. They can laugh while they spend time looking for the right card for you. Let them know that it's all right to be a clown at times, and to share tears at other times. We must live what we feel in order to heal.

If you and your team follow the principles and suggestions provided here, you'll empower yourselves and make a winning team. You won't be immortal, but you'll be winners because you'll be living fully. In the next chapter, we'll talk about healing and wholeness, and the difference between being *healed* and being *cured*. Throughout the rest of the book, and throughout your illness and your healing, don't forget that empowered teams draw their strength from faith, hope, and love—and that the greatest of these is love.

❧

CHAPTER 2

Healing and How It Happens

Bernie: Spring was in the air, and John Florio was planning to retire. John had worked hard all his life as a commercial landscaper, planting thousands of bulbs, plants, and trees, and creating a beautiful world for all to enjoy. He was best known for surrounding office buildings with flowers that made everyone's workday a little easier and a lot more lovely. But that year, as John planned to give up his work, he developed a burning sensation in his stomach. At first he took antacids; when the distress continued, he saw his physician.

Suspecting an ulcer due to John's depression and stress over his impending retirement, the doctor ordered a series of gastrointestinal x-rays and prescribed stronger medication, which did nothing to relieve John's symptoms. Further tests revealed an enlarging ulcer, and a biopsy confirmed that he had a carcinoma of the stomach.

It was at this point that John came to my office. Knowing the seriousness of the situation, I said: "John, I have a week's vacation coming up, but I don't want to delay your operation, so let's get you right into the hospital."

"You forgot something," John said.

"What's that?"

"It's springtime. I'm going home to make the world beautiful. When I'm done, I'll return for the operation."

So I went on vacation. After I returned, several more weeks passed before John reappeared at my office to tell me that he was ready for the operation. He was admitted to the hospital, and I performed the surgery. I found a large malignant tumor that couldn't be completely removed. The next morning I sat down at his bedside.

"John, I couldn't remove all the cancer," I explained. "You need more treatment—possibly chemotherapy and radiation."

"You forgot something," John said.

"What did I forget?"

"It's still spring. I don't have time for your treatment. I'm going home to make the world beautiful. If I die, I'll have left something wonderful behind."

I didn't argue with him, and neither did his family. John went home and never returned for his scheduled office visits.

Four years later, I came into the office and noticed John's chart in one of the examining room racks. I turned to my nurse: "Anne, you have the wrong chart—John Florio is dead. We must have two patients by the same name. Get me the correct chart."

"Why don't you open the door?" she suggested.

So I did, and there in the examining room sat John.

"Hi, Doc," he said. "I have a hernia from lifting boulders in my landscape business."

We fixed his hernia on an outpatient basis because John wanted no part of hospitals. And to my amazement, there was no sign of cancer anywhere in his body.

Over the years I treated John for a variety of other aches and pains related to his work, and eventually I began to spend time with him outside the office. He became my teacher, showing me how glorious the world is when you know how to look at it. He taught me to see tiny flowers and colors in places I'd never looked before. When I was with John, I felt like an extraterrestrial who was seeing the planet for the first time. To this day, I collect flowers as I jog or bike. I bring them home to plant in my yard, where they remind me of John and his lessons about seeing beauty everywhere.

When John was in his 90s, his wife became ill and they moved into a nursing home together. John continued gardening and making the world beautiful. He lived to be 94, with no sign of his cancer ever returning. In his last years, John wrote an autobiography in which he said, "I always hope I'll die working in my garden."

He did, because the *world* was his garden.

What Healing Is

Healing is connected to living and loving. It's the experience of wholeness, or holiness. It's being as one with life and our Creator. Curing, on the other hand, refers to the physical body. Being cured means overcoming a disease and, for the time being, postponing death.

But doctors can't cure every disease, and ultimately, you can't avoid death. You can, however, be sure that you don't miss the chance to live. You can always heal your life, because you're always capable of loving and living more fully. Sometimes the by-product of healing your life is being cured. A 90-year-old patient we treated was so full of life that she was, in her words, "too busy to die." The will to live is a powerful force.

Some spiritual traditions view the moment of birth as a passage from a state of wholeness and knowledge to a state of forgetting. In this view of the world, we spend the rest of our lives searching for wholeness and knowledge, wellness and health—the balance and harmony we lost when we were born. If our wholeness is interrupted, then our health suffers, and we need to find a way to restore our sense of meaning. When we move in the direction of that meaning, we're healing.

This is not a new concept. The Hebrew word *shalom* is usually translated as "peace," or "hello" and "good-bye." But *shalom* also means "wholeness." In Hebrew, the question, "How are you doing?" is derived from *shalom,* so although the speaker may not be aware of it, he or she is actually asking, "How is your wholeness?"

Sometimes healing brings a cure or a full restoration of health, but it's important to recognize that healing isn't a single destination point; it's a path that moves us toward balance. Many people have had afflictions that can't be cured, but they're still whole—think, for example, of Helen Keller.

Bernie: To heal, or to be whole, you must attain peace of mind, but that's a very difficult state to achieve in today's society. In my next life, I plan to live as far away from electricity as possible—far from artificial power and Palm Pilots, shopping lists and answering machines. I'll just stoke the fire when it dies down and go hunt for breakfast with the guys, then come home and play with my children and pets. In the afternoon, I'll hunt some more, nap, teach the kids to catch game, eat, tell stories around the fire, and then go to sleep. I'll have no credit cards or bills and no schedule to keep, and by doing nothing I'll accomplish everything.

The world we live in is much more difficult. Most of us live with a sense of discomfort that Carl Jung called a "gnawing unrest." The unrest actually isn't a bad thing to feel, given the world we find ourselves in. Just as pain protects us, our unrest warns us that something is wrong or missing in these lives of ours, which are dominated by artificiality and too-busy schedules.

To find the peace that heals, you have to identify the source of your unrest. You may need to ask yourself: "Why am I feeling this way? What's affecting me? What do I need to change in my life?" Then, the most important question becomes: "What will I do with this information?" We can let our busyness or our past unhappy experiences burden us, and we can continue to feel guilt, shame, blame, resentment, and bitterness—or we can make use of the heat and energy generated by those feelings. It may be difficult to leave the negative emotions and to move to a place of understanding, loving, and forgiving, but it's possible.

We all have the power within us to heal ourselves. None of us has to be a lifelong victim, always feeling guilty or making excuses for being unable to be healed or cured. Think about how it feels to be bitter, resentful, and depressed, and imagine what those feelings can do to your body and health. In contrast, recall a time when you experienced appropriate anger over something that happened to you. That kind of emotion generates energy and leads you into action. After you've experienced appropriate anger, you can move on to understanding and feelings of forgiveness and love for yourself and others, no matter what's been done. If you want true freedom and healing, learn to love the unlovable and forgive the unforgivable.

It's been proven that the immune function and cortisol (a steroid hormone that regulates blood pressure and metabolism) levels of actors are altered by the roles they perform. They're only acting, but you're living your life—so imagine the effect your psychology can have on your physiology. Know that your attitude, emotions, and feelings *are* your chemistry.

More evidence of this phenomenon was uncovered in another scientific investigation, the *Ohio Longitudinal Study,* which revealed that people with positive attitudes about the future live, on average, seven and a half years longer than those who aren't optimistic. In fact, attitude proved to be a more significant factor in longevity than exercise or smoking. More and more studies are revealing that compassion and positive relationships lead to longer survival rates in people who have AIDS and cancer, and are show-ing that relationships affect the immune system and a tumor's ability to develop new blood vessels. So John Florio's story is truly about self-induced healing, not a spontaneous remission.

If you want to be on a healing path, you have to be cognizant of your beliefs about yourself and the world. *You* define what's stressful and what's just one of life's redirections. So if you choose to view your life as a learning process, then you'll experience the "stressful" events differently. You'll be able to stop seeing things as either good or bad, and start appreciating them as opportunities to learn to deal with difficulties—maybe you'll even see them as having potential future benefits.

We know of a 93-year-old blind woman whose husband died. The woman was admitted to an assisted-living facility, and as she was being wheeled in, she said, "Oh, what a beautiful place." The attendant pointed out that she was blind and asked how she could say that her new home was beautiful.

"I have a choice about how I see the world," the woman answered, "and I choose to see it as beautiful."

Bernie: I often talk about 90-year-olds when I tell sto-ries about people who have found peace. The reason is simple: When you make it to 90, you've already lived through all of the things that the rest of us still fear. I've often asked my 90-year-old patients to join our support group as therapists, because they can help others survive what they've already lived through. When I asked one sup-port group what they feared, a woman in her 90s thought awhile before answering: "Driving on the parkway at night." When that's all you fear, you're ready to be a teacher and help others survive their life-threatening situations.

Sometimes younger folks can be teachers, too. I was helped by a 78-year-old woman I met while I was jogging on an exercise trail in our town. The woman stopped me to tell me how lucky I was to be able to run while she had trouble walking. That changed my day. I'd been so focused on the trouble I was having completing enough miles to prepare for a marathon I wanted to run, but this woman reminded me that I need to be aware of what I have to be grateful for each day.

When it comes to finding a teacher, age is not the issue. Our family dog is only four, but he teaches our support group. When I bring him to meetings, he shows us how to make noise and display emotion when we want something. Children will teach you the same lesson, until they start to grow up, internalize feelings, and learn to "behave" to avoid troubling people. The children who learn these behavior lessons well are more likely to develop cancer as adults. If they live to reach 90, you can be sure that they dumped the lessons about so-called good behavior along the way.

Of course, not all 90-year-olds are perfect. My mom is in her 90s and still finds time to worry about the things that disturb her peace or threaten people she loves. We're all human, and we all have some struggles to find peace—even at 90—but in general we get better at it with time.

Cautions about Healing

Bernie: One word of warning from my personal experience: Sometimes when we're ill, the problem isn't stress or gnawing unrest. Sometimes disease is a simple and straightforward physical problem that may be cured easily, even without healing.

Some years ago I began suffering from fatigue and daily headaches. Every day I'd think about what was happening in my life and ask questions about what might be causing my symptoms. I analyzed and meditated and tried to figure out where my life needed healing. I asked myself:

"What's making me feel ill? What do I need to change?" I wondered if it could be my travel schedule, relationships, or work. I thought about it for a couple of weeks, but got no relief. No matter what I did, the fatigue and headaches persisted. Finally, I noticed a rash on my leg and realized I had Lyme disease. I started taking antibiotics, and within a day the fatigue and headaches were gone. The lesson is obvious: Sometimes symptoms are due solely to physical disease. You may be able to see a doctor, get treatment, and be cured . . . and not be neurotic like me.

One final caution on the subject of healing: Don't fall into the trap of blaming yourself for your illness. People are sometimes tempted to do this when they learn that certain beliefs and actions can promote healing. If you find that you're unable to cure your disease, you may be tempted to view your illness as a personal defeat. That's certainly not our view. We don't blame anyone for illness, and we don't believe that illness is punishment inflicted by our Creator.

Over the years, we've sometimes been accused of setting people up for failure. Some of our critics have said that when we talk about making healing choices, we're in effect saying that people who are ill have only themselves to blame. This is simply a misunderstanding of our message about healing. Being responsible for yourself and participating in your treatment doesn't mean that you must feel guilty and accept blame for your illness. If you want to heal, the last thing you should do is view your disease as a punishment.

Think, for example, about insomnia. It's no secret that restful sleep promotes healing, but it would be absurd to blame an insomniac for refusing to fall asleep. It would be ridiculous to argue that insomniacs who want to be cured should simply stop tossing and turning and just fall asleep. We do maintain that with the help of a sleep specialist, an insomniac can be trained to relax and may be able to increase the amount of rest he or she gets. At the same time, we know that learning to relax is difficult, and that some patients may progress slowly even with a competent coach. When we point out that some changes lead to healing and may result in cures, we're not criticizing people who aren't willing or able to make those changes in their lives. If you blame the insomniac or the man suffering chronic pain or the woman with cancer, you're missing the point of healing.

We know that your behavior, and your response to illness, is influenced by whether you've been loved and whether you're able to love yourself now. We see you as a divine child, and we're here to love and accept you and your choices. We hope that you'll be able to love and accept yourself no matter what your parents, teachers, and religious instructors may have taught you in the past.

Healing Actions and Healing Beliefs

What actions can you take to promote the flow of love, wholeness, and well-being in your life? Surprisingly, healing actions are easier to perform than unhealing ones. For instance, you may have difficulty expressing your feelings and standing up for yourself, and based upon your past experiences, you might think that it's easier to be stoic or simply to be quiet. Your life is stored within you, but the reality is, it takes less energy to express your feelings than to suppress them—and it's healthier. It may be difficult to express your feelings the first few times you try, but once you get in the habit, you'll see how much easier it is. Asking for what you want may be hard when it hasn't been part of your experience, but it's less strenuous than suffering in silence. Likewise, forgiving people who do you wrong is easier than holding on to your resentment in the long run, and it frees you from a lifetime of unhappiness.

Some healing actions are major projects that will require dedicated work on your part. Others are everyday actions—things you may do routinely but don't think of as healing. Every time you forgive someone, express your feelings, pay attention to your body and your intuition, or experience or express gratitude, you're performing a healing action. When you decide to question medical advice rather than blindly accept it, or when you ask about the purpose and efficacy of a medical treatment your doctor recommends, you're again walking down the healing path.

Here is a list of healing actions for you to consider. Think of this list as a foundation, and as you work on healing, adapt it to build your own framework upon. Write us, or better, e-mail us at **healing@bedscapes.com** so that we can share your ideas and help other people with their healing.

1. Examine your beliefs. Your beliefs play a major role in determining what happens to you. By *beliefs,* we mean your spiritual understanding as well as your common, everyday assumptions about yourself and your life. You live what you believe—your beliefs are your biology.

Spiritual beliefs can be healing beliefs, especially if you can turn your troubles over to God or some other higher power. If you've ever tried this, you probably know that it creates inner peace, but you may not realize how much that peace enhances your ability to heal. Studies show that people who view God or religion as a resource live longer, healthier lives. The findings hold true for many different religions and spiritual practices: Meditation, imagery, healing touch, prayer, and other spiritual or faith-based resources have all been shown to promote healing.

> **Bernie:** As much as religion can help you heal, it can also be a hindrance. Religious beliefs become a burden when they make you feel less loved and less loving. Authoritarian religions can promote destructive myths and turn people away from healing paths, while fundamentalist religions can cause a lot of grief, especially when they make the believers feel guilty and teach that people outside the faith are evil or satanic. A minister in Tupelo, Mississippi, labeled me "satanic" because I teach meditation

and the use of healing imagery. The minister warned his followers against these practices because, he argued, when we close our eyes, Satan can appear and take control of our images.

I talked with that minister and told him I wasn't saying anything that Jesus hadn't said. I reminded him of the message that Jesus shared with his disciples when they questioned him about the blind man. The disciples asked whose sin had led to the man being punished with blindness, but Jesus answered that the issue was not sinning but manifesting God's work. Jesus healed the blind man by telling him, "Thy faith has saved thee." The message is not a mechanical message, such as "Rise up and walk," but a healing message. The man's faith resulted in his healing, and a *by-product* of healing was the return of his vision.

If your religious beliefs don't focus on forgiveness, or if you believe in a god who punishes individuals, then your spiritual life isn't likely to help you to heal. If you view your illness as a punishment for your sins, then you may even feel you don't deserve to be healed. Spiritual traditions that emphasize forgiveness and mercy along with justice are obviously much better for your health. Your beliefs can help you heal if you view illness as a teacher, a gift from which you can learn something, or simply lost health that needs restoring. When we lose our car keys, we don't say that God wants us to walk home. So when we lose our health, why would we assume that God wants us to be sick?

Illness is a wonderful opportunity to reexamine your beliefs—especially your beliefs about being worthwhile and entitled to love. You'd be amazed to know how many people are walking around in the world convinced that they're inferior. If you're one of them, then you have a lot of company—even some of our most admired celebrities have really low opinions of themselves. Please accept our gift of a new belief system that says: *You're not inferior. You're not a problem, despite what the authorities in your life may have told you. You're a child of God.* Even if you're an atheist, it's our belief that you're nonetheless of divine origin. We're all made of the same creative energy, and we all deserve to be treated with love and dignity.

Bernie: Our beliefs don't all come from religion or spiritual training. Some beliefs come to us as family attitudes or assumptions. Whenever my family encountered trouble, my mother would say, "Something good will come of this," because she viewed difficulties as God's way of redirecting us toward something better. Some of us are fortunate enough to grow up with parents who have a healthy view of life, where intuition is honored and decisions are not based on "What do you think I should do?" but rather on "What are you feeling?" or "What will make you happy?"

In my talks, I used to ask people what mottoes they lived by. Some of the healthy mottoes were: "Troubles are God's way of redirecting you." "When you have to make a decision, do what makes you happy." "Life is like a baseball game—it isn't over until the last out." "The purpose of money is to make life easier for people."

One night, a man who heard my talk said, "You should also ask what mottoes people are dying by." So I asked that question, and people replied: "Don't be too happy—every happy day is followed by a sad day." "Something good is always followed by something bad." "Life is like a football game—you lose when time runs out." "There's something wrong with me, and everything bad that happens to me is my own fault." "The purpose of money is to measure success."

As your first healing action, examine the mottoes and beliefs you were taught by your family, your religion, and your teachers. Were you taught that you're divine? That you deserve love? That your feelings are important and that they should be expressed? If you discover that you were raised with mottoes to *die* by, you can try to adopt some new mottoes to *live* by. You can make a choice about what to believe. You can adopt these healing beliefs:

- Love is what matters—and the more you give, the more you'll receive (although true love is given without condition).

- You're entitled to love—you were born 100-percent lovable, and nothing you've ever done or ever will do can change that. Look at your baby pictures to see the truth in this.

- You're entitled to express your feelings.

- Laughter and joy are choices that are always available.

- Every moment is an opportunity for a new beginning.

- You can always move toward wholeness and healing.

- Forgiveness is a gift you give to yourself.

2. Love and let yourself be loved. Giving and receiving love is a critical part of healing. Surprisingly, most of us are better at giving than receiving. We have so many underachievers that we need a new diagnosis—RDD, or **R**eceiving **D**eficit **D**isorder. Unfortunately, there's no simple fix for RDD; no pill or medical procedure corrects this condition. To overcome RDD, you have to reexamine your beliefs about being entitled to love. Then you have to practice accepting even small gestures of love that come your way. You may be surprised at how abundant these are once you begin to notice and welcome them. Over time, receiving love can become a new habit in your life.

Learning to give and receive love isn't easy work if you weren't brought up in a loving home, but it's essential because love and health are inseparable. One study of Harvard students provides a striking demonstration of the link between loving and health: Students who described their parents as caring and loving had surprisingly good health in the 35 years after their graduation. It didn't matter whether the parents divorced or stayed married, drank or smoked. As long as the students felt their parents were "caring and loving," they had only a 28-percent chance of suffering a major illness in those 35 years. By contrast, of the students who said that their parents were not caring and loving, 98 percent suffered a major illness within 35 years of graduating from college.

Another study showed that monkeys separated from their mothers for the first seven months of their lives became alcoholics when they were later given the opportunity to drink, while those who weren't separated didn't imbibe.

As important as parental love is, it's perhaps even more important that you love yourself. When you're able to do this, you won't behave in destructive ways or become addicted in your search for the feeling of being loved. If you have trouble acting as if you love yourself, then try treating yourself the way a loving grandparent would treat you. When you re-parent yourself and find self-love, you'll heal your life.

3. Learn from your illness. Just as you can learn about the source of your pain by describing it, you can learn about your life by analyzing your experience with illness. You can ask yourself what the practical consequences of your disease are, and what this might tell you about your life. Ask what your disease has accomplished for you that you could achieve in other, more healthy ways. If you're often ill on Monday, then perhaps your feelings about your job are making you sick and you need to think about finding employment elsewhere—before you become one of the many people who has a heart attack or commits suicide on the first day of the workweek.

To learn from your illness, you can ask what it is that's happened in your life that may have made you vulnerable or susceptible at this time. What path do you need to follow to change and heal? What makes you feel alive? What gives your life meaning? What unconscious destructive script might you be following? What are your psychological genetics—what's your family psychological inheritance? What fears or inadequacies did you learn from your parents? What did they teach you that may be killing you? What are you not saying or not willing to feel? You came into the world with a life stored within you—and that life needs to be brought forth if you want to heal. Again, what you keep sealed within you can kill you—literally.

As you reflect on these questions, remember to avoid falling into the trap of blaming yourself for your illness. This is about changing your life or your attitude about your life, not about finding someone or something to blame.

4. Join a support group. You'll need help as you do the work of examining your beliefs, learning from your illness, and transforming your life. Support groups can offer the help that family members and friends may not be able to give. Choose your support group carefully, though. Some are dominated by whining and "poor me" victim attitudes. You'll want to find a group that focuses on survival behavior and healing. If you find one with people who have had experiences similar to yours, you'll find mentors and role models and will experience a new sense of hope. When you join a support group, you become a member of a new and healthy family.

5. Ask for what you want. We talked in Chapter 1 about letting people know what you need. This is important enough that it belongs on every list of healing actions.

6. Say no when you don't want to do something. Saying no to others is sometimes really a way of saying yes to yourself. You help yourself heal when you say no to treatments that don't make sense to you, intrusions on your personal space and privacy, and other people's negative thinking and worrying.

7. Say yes when that's what you're feeling. This is often left out in assertiveness training. Saying no is important, but if you're really empowered, you can also say yes, for it's a way of letting love and care into your life. You want to be able to say yes to offers of the kind of help you want, to expressions of love and kindness, to life, and even to death when it's the right time for you to let go.

8. Insist on being treated as a human being. You're not a diagnosis or a room number. You can make this point playfully when you create and use Vital Signs (see Chapter 5) and do the healing activities that your team prescribes and that you choose from the "Healing Ways" (Part III) section in this book. You show that you're on a healing path when you say yes to taking control of your own healing, and no to the voices in your head that provide abundant excuses for postponing activities that can help you heal.

9. Laugh. Go for the belly laugh. or what Norman Cousins called "internal jogging." Laughing is great aerobic exercise, and it helps strengthen the immune system. When you don't feel able to laugh, try smiling. Recent research shows that the simple muscular act of smiling—even forced smiling—convinces your brain you're experiencing something pleasurable. When your brain thinks you're happy, you'll feel better. If you behave like a child again, laughter will follow.

10. Hug. Hug anyone and everyone you can. But ask permission, and respect the fact that some people have been abused physically and sexually, or they simply may not want to be touched.

11. Forgive. If you want to heal, you have to forgive yourself and others—significant others, those outside your intimate circle, and everyone else—over and over and over and over again.

Forgiveness means letting go of the hurt. You forgive from your psyche, but more important you forgive from your body by not holding on to your anger and bitterness. This doesn't mean that you accept behavior that's unhealthy for you, it simply means that you won't hold on to the hurt.

Yosaif: If you find that you can't entirely forgive someone who has wronged you, use a technique my friend Bahira recommends: Try viewing forgiveness as an onion—peel back a layer of forgiveness now, and forgive more as time goes on. If you want to feel rejuvenated, try forgiving everyone just before you go to sleep. Forgive anyone who consciously or unconsciously didn't support your well-being during the day. If you can't forgive entirely, just peel back one more layer of forgiveness. You'll sleep better, dream better, and wake up more refreshed and renewed.

12. Give yourself some Sabbath or white-room time. Give yourself time to meditate, pray, heal, or simply to *be*. Talk to your body and visualize it healing frequently throughout the day. Make sure you take the time to do things you enjoy. You're in the healthiest possible emotional and physical state when you're doing something that makes you lose track of time. In that state, you're ageless, in a trance, and free of all afflictions. When you do something you love that much, you're giving a gift to your body and mind.

Think back to times when you've had this experience. Now recall times when you were feeling guilt, shame, or blame. You can probably feel the reaction in your body that occurs simply by remembering those different types of experiences. Think about how you're spending your lifetime, because what you experience and what you feel affects your ability to heal—both psychologically and physically.

❦

You can add other healing actions to this list, but be careful how you view them. Don't be discouraged if you can't do everything on your list or if you fail to do things perfectly. You don't have to do everything, and you don't have to do anything perfectly. Your goal isn't perfection, it's healing, and healing means living and loving fully. Healing means that you don't let disease become your life, and you don't live a role prescribed by your illness or other people's expectations. You neither deny your illness nor resign yourself to it—you accept it and empower yourself to heal in its presence. You put your energy into actions that bring forth your true, authentic self. This is hard work, but it's possible. Many people have done it, and you can, too. You can live fully in the presence of disease if you have a strategy or game plan.

In the rest of this book, we'll give you practical suggestions about how you can (1) turn your environment into a sacred healing space, (2) turn visits into healing encounters, and (3) build and nurture your own healing team.

〜

CHAPTER 3

Preparing for a Healthy Hospitalization

The words *healthy hospitalization* may sound like an oxymoron. How can hospitalization be healthy? The truth is that any hospitalization we *survive* should be considered healthy, but there's more to it than that: We want people to experience true healing while in the hospital.

The dictionary defines a patient as "a person who is under medical or surgical treatment." That much is okay, but it goes on to say that a patient is "a sufferer or victim." The word *patient* is derived from a Latin word meaning "to undergo, suffer, bear." To *be patient* means to "bear annoyance, pain, etc., without complaint or anger." Synonyms are "invalid," "uncomplaining," "long-suffering," and "forbearing."

All of this suffering and forbearing pretty much describes what's expected of us when we become patients. In the hospital we're expected to be very, very patient. The problem is that this isn't a good way to recover from illness. Studies show that people identified by nurses as "difficult" patients have better survival statistics than the "good" patients.

In other words, to prepare for a healthy hospitalization, you don't need to prepare to be a good patient. That won't help you heal. You need to find a way out of the "submissive sufferer" role and a way into a more active one in which you can orchestrate your own healing. Since our language has no good word for this type of role, we've coined the term *respant*. We define a respant as "a responsible participant—someone willing to take responsibility for his or her own life."

It may seem strange to talk about being a participant in your own care, because we're taught to think that the details of our treatment are none of our business. This is especially true in a hospital—everything about the hospital experience encourages you to believe that you have no choice but to submit to your situation exactly as it is. But the truth is that you have a lot of choices, and as a respant, you'll make decisions about your care at every step in your journey.

In this chapter, we'll talk about the important decisions you can make before you enter the hospital.

Choosing a Hospital

The most important step in your preparation is deciding whether hospitalization is the best course for you—maybe you'd do better with outpatient procedures or other forms of treatment. Don't make this decision based on fear; instead, rely on the medical information you receive and your feelings about what's right for you.

If your physician doesn't present options when he or she recommends hospitalization, ask why. If the timing and other details of your stay are dictated by your doctor's schedule or your insurance company's policy, then act like a respant—speak up and let everyone know that *you* have a schedule, too. Remember that there are many doctors and hospitals available. If the problem turns out to be your insurance company, don't hesitate to use a lawyer to express your needs and to insist on getting appropriate care.

It's usually preferable to choose a hospital near your support team so they can visit and act as your empowering advocates when you need them. If you need specialized care and have to be hospitalized at a distance, consider taking someone with you and having them stay at a nearby hotel. If the hospital is local but your family isn't, ask someone to house-sit for you while you're hospitalized. They can overfeed the pets, get the mail, and do other housekeeping chores for you.

When you're preparing for an elective hospitalization, you can choose a hospital that's right for you in terms of size, distance from home, follow-up care, reputation, and the attitude of the staff. If you come from a small town, some major medical centers located in large cities can be overwhelming and depersonalizing. In a large hospital, you can easily become a number rather than an individual to the staff. So, if you choose a large medical center, see if you can get a patient advocate assigned to you.

Bernie: The attitude of the medical staff can make an enormous difference in your convalescence. When my father-in-law became quadriplegic due to a fall, we cared for him at home for as long as we could. When we needed help, we took him to a nursing home where he soon developed abdominal pain and vomiting. He underwent various tests, but nothing revealed the cause of his illness. It was obvious, though, that he was dying.

At about that time, a new nursing home was built near our home. We moved him there so that we could spend more time with him in the last days of his life. His insurance company didn't approve the transfer, so I became responsible for his medical expenses.

The day after the move, he was sitting up—free of pain. The next day he was able to eat without vomiting. By the fourth day it was clear that he wasn't dying anytime soon, and I was still paying all the bills. I asked him, "How come you're not dying anymore?" He replied, "They were tired of caring for me in the other nursing home. I was dying to make them happy."

He lived for several more years, and the insurance company resumed paying his medical bills (thank God) until he died quietly and naturally one night, by his own choice, at the age of 97.

People are especially vulnerable to illness or accident when they're going through major changes: a divorce, the death of a loved one, the loss of a job, or a move to a new community. The more of these changes you're experiencing, the more likely you are to become sick or injured. If you need to be hospitalized in the midst of these events, don't go it alone. Make sure you maintain contact with people you know and care about and who care about you.

If you have a choice about the length of your stay, you may choose outpatient or short-term care to avoid the risks and complications of hospitalization. Outpatient treatment may be the right choice if you have a lot of support from family and friends or if you're able to hire private-duty nurses and home-health aides. Convalescent-care facilities are another option. The important point is that you don't neglect yourself or try to act heroic by caring for yourself—that will just hinder your recovery.

You may be tempted to choose a short stay so that you can return home to take care of your usual concerns, such as mail, pets, yard, house, children, spouse, and whatever else is on your mind or schedule. However, if you'll need follow-up care and you don't have family or friends to provide transportation or nurse you at home, then don't be in a hurry to leave the hospital. You may be better off remaining there for a while, especially if you're the type of person who's unaccustomed to taking time to care for yourself. You can ask a neighbor to pick up your mail, sort it, and bring it to you in the hospital, and you can hire someone to keep an eye on your home if your team is unavailable for this task. Once you start planning, you'll find that there are solutions to every problem if you just ask for help. You may be amazed by how smoothly things run at home when your family members have to do for themselves all the things you normally take care of.

Preparing to Enter the Hospital

Think of your upcoming experience as a trip to a foreign country. Using this book as a traveler's guide, prepare for a visit to the land of health and healing. Talk to the natives (those who have been through this before) ahead of time, consult a travel agent (medical experts, both mainstream and holistic), and pack what you'll need. Learn the language before you leave home (the language is medical terminology, and learning it can help demystify your experience). Find out as much as you can about what the experience will be like, and let everyone know what you're feeling and experiencing and what you need to heal.

As we said in Chapter 1, healing is a team sport. You need a healing team to ensure that you'll be surrounded by people who care about you and who can act as your empowering advocates throughout your healing journey. If you form your team before you enter the hospital, then they can help you with your prehospitalization preparations. You'll want people on the team who can support the decisions you make, so you need to let them know what to expect when you ask them to sign on. Be explicit—tell them that you're a respant and you intend to be active in making medical choices. Explain your beliefs about healing, what kinds of attitudes you want to be surrounded by, and how assertive you intend to be with health-care professionals. Remember that your preferences may change during different phases of your journey.

If you have a significant other, he or she can be the coach or conductor of your team. If you don't, then it will probably be an especially challenging time for you—you may be feeling scared and very much alone, and these feelings are natural and understandable. You can ask a family member or friend to lead your team, or you can do it yourself. Remember that whatever your situation, you're entitled to love and caring. Illness is a challenge, but it's also an opportunity to reach out for the love and support you need.

We know many people without significant others who called on friends for assistance and were surprised and moved to see how everyone responded. A physician friend of ours noted that some people he knew quite well backed away from him when he was a "wounded healer," while others he hadn't been close to before stepped forward with love and care. Another friend facing hospitalization without a significant other at his side was touched by a number of people who offered to transport him to and from the hospital and who signed up to provide support on different days during his convalescence. Several of the people who volunteered said it was a kind of payback for the many times over the years that he'd been there for them.

Team-building can be a great experience for you, and what your friends learn from the experience may be a gift to them. Be aware, though, that some people won't be comfortable joining your healing team, which is their right. Those who are comfortable will step forward; those who aren't will opt out. The group that emerges through this process is usually exactly the right one for your needs.

Your family and friends may want to organize themselves into a "healing tag team" to look after your well-being before, during, and after your hospitalization. This will be especially important when you make your transition back home (or to another facility) to complete your convalescence. A tag team works together to make sure that you have continual support. This approach also provides respite for those who are caring for you.

The tag-team strategy requires a visiting schedule. The Internet is a simple and effective tool that each visitor can use to let others know what needs to be done and what things you need brought to you. Before you're hospitalized, you or someone on the team can put together an e-mail list that will let your friends know how you're doing and what your up-to-the-minute needs are. A Website (or a page on an existing site) is a fancier tool, but an e-mail list works fine as a simple, easy method to communicate:

- a visiting schedule that can be posted and updated;

- a list of items you need brought to you by visitors;

- a list of errands you need run or calls you need made on your behalf;

- a spot for loving, healing messages that can be printed out and brought to your bedside; and

- suggestions for healthy foods and snacks to bring, including easy-to-prepare recipes.

You might want to get your team together for a prehospitalization Vital Signs party. This is a gathering that provides you with love and support while your teammates have fun sharing healing wisdom, creating Vital Signs and healing objects, and sampling healing music for you to bring to the hospital and back home for your convalescence.

These gatherings are actually part of your healing journey and a form of medicine, because the desire, intention, and determination of your loved ones can change you. You don't have to wait for the clinical research on this—we know that people who participate in healing conclaves have stronger immune-system responses.

These gatherings are also important for the people who care about you. While they're painting, embroidering, and sewing, they're also tapping in to the energy of healing. By being actively involved in the preparations, they can overcome their own sense of helplessness and the feeling of powerlessness that people often experience when they surrender their loved one to the care of a hospital.

The Vital Signs you create are communication tools. They're signs that you'll hang on your door or in your room to let people know how best to help you heal. (You'll find coaching tips on creating and using Vital Signs in Chapter 5.) Some Vital Signs we've seen deliver a wide range of messages:

- Gone Fishin'—back in 15 minutes.

- Thank you for being here!

- Speak to my spirit, not my diagnosis.

If you approach it with total abandon, writing Vital Signs can be a joyful experience. Work together with your team to think up 20, 50, even 100 signs. Don't censor yourselves—indulge in exaggeration, outrageousness, and playfulness. This is a time to be expressive and creative. Later you can edit your signs and choose which ones to actually bring to the hospital.

People at your Vital Signs party can also create Visitor Cards, which your visitors will use when they arrive and find you resting, or when your Vital Sign indicates that you prefer being alone at that moment. Your visitors can write loving messages for you and leave the card at the nurses' station. (See Chapter 6 for more hints on creating these cards.)

While you're working with your team, you're the only judge of propriety, and you set the standard of appropriateness. The same rule applies when you're creating healing objects and other props to make a healing place out of your hospital room and wherever else you'll be convalescing. People sometimes feel that they have to be serious and somber about healing, but your healing can have whatever spirit you want. Your signs and objects can be playful if that feels right to you.

Know that you can indulge in as much lighthearted, childlike humor as you desire, but we suggest avoiding humor relating to denial and pretense. Humor becomes unhealthy when it suppresses the expression of important feelings, or when it wastes an opportunity for sharing. Unhealthy humor can support a pretense that nothing is wrong and there's no reason to worry. Sometimes people use it as a foundation for an unstated mutual conspiracy in which a patient, for the sake of a loved one, agrees to pretend that illness doesn't exist. This places a burden on the patient and interferes with honest communication.

Healthy humor is playful, fun, and honest. It promotes healing by providing an escape valve that relieves fear, tension, and stress. Shared laughs that grow out of healthy humor can help send you giggling your way out of the hospital in record time. So when you have a bladder problem, you can tell the nurse that you were just following directions—the sign in the corridor said "Wet Floor" and you did. Or, when you're asked to sign in, write *in* on the paper they hand you.

Other Ways to Prepare

Guided visualization. Your team can help with a lot of your preparation, but there are some jobs they can't do for you. Guided visualization is one proven healing technique that you must practice yourself.

Studies have revealed that guided visualization can reduce pain and anxiety, speed healing, and send you home sooner. The technique is similar to what athletes and performers do when they imagine success before the whistle blows or the curtain rises. In guided visualization, you'll prepare for successful treatment by "seeing" the outcome you want. You may already be using a negative form of guided visualization: If you spend time dwelling on your worst fears and worries, then you're increasing the chances that you'll have exactly the kinds of side effects and complications you dread.

To prepare for a successful treatment, find a quiet, comfortable place and put on some relaxing music. You may use a prepared audiotape or one you've created yourself, or do without it if you prefer. Then picture yourself going to the hospital, being admitted, meeting caring people, and having your procedure performed or receiving treatment with no complications. Next, visualize yourself awakening comfortable and hungry, recovering rapidly and going home well. If you do this several times a day, your mind and body will be programmed to experience the treatment or procedure without fear and worry. If you're having surgery, you can prepare a tape for the staff to play in the operating room during the procedure; or, as Yosaif did, you can write out your own healing message for yourself and ask the O.R. staff to read it to you while you're under anesthesia.

Guided visualization works because your body doesn't know the difference between the real thing and what you visualize. By the time you have your procedure, your body will think that it has already had many successful procedures. You've trained it to anticipate—and to work toward—the outcome you want.

Continue this work in the hospital and after your treatment to help you heal and recover faster. To give yourself the privacy you'll need, hang one of your Vital Signs and close your hospital-room door. The hospital staff can empty the wastebasket and take your temperature later—meanwhile, you're busy healing.

If you need help with your visualization, find an imagery therapist or hypnotherapist to make a tape for you. If you're a visual person, you'll need a tape that directs you to picture everything. If you're auditory, tactile, or olfactory, you'll want to include in your exercises sounds, sensations, and aromas that you're sensitive to and that you expect will help in your healing.

For more details about guided-visualization tapes geared toward specific concerns, such as controlling bleeding or other physiological functions, see the Exceptional Cancer Patients (ECaP) Website at **www.ecap-online.org.**

Spontaneous drawings. Before you're admitted, draw a picture of yourself in the operating room or hospital receiving treatment. You don't have to be an artist—a simple drawing with crayons will do. You're not being graded, and you can't do it wrong. Anything you draw will work, because pictures inevitably reveal intuitive wisdom and expectations, showing the complications and benefits you expect from your hospitalization. With help, you can analyze your drawings and then address issues before they become problems. For example, if you draw a picture that doesn't include your doctor and your family, then you might need to make sure that these important people are more fully involved in your hospitalization. If your picture is drawn all in black, you might need to think over your feelings about your illness and your upcoming hospitalization. What you learn from your drawing can help you create a healthy guided-visualization exercise.

Pictures are an invaluable tool for understanding children, too. If you're preparing for a child's hospitalization, plan to bring along a pad of paper and crayons for spontaneous artwork, as well as specific, directed drawings. Sometimes it's best not to tell the child that you're using the drawings to analyze feelings, because he or she may resist drawing for that purpose. If the child does agree to draw, his or her mood will be revealed in the colors and subjects he or she chooses. Drawings can also reveal anatomical clues that a physician may not be aware of and that might be useful in making the correct diagnosis and choosing an appropriate treatment. (Further details about how to learn from drawings are available on the ECaP Website.)

Dreams can provide similar insight into your illness and your body's potential response to the treatments you're considering. But remember that mind and body communicate through symbols, not words. When you understand this, you can use your intuitive and unconscious energy and wisdom to guide your healing process. You may need help understanding your dreams, so you may want to consult a therapist or one of the many books available on exploring dreams.

Learn from the experience of others. You don't have to learn everything the hard way—that is, through your own pain and suffering. You can learn from the wisdom of sages, and you might as well begin before you go into the hospital.

We're all wounded, and most of us have been informed, but not really *educated,* about life. We're given facts, but we're not taught how to deal with our wounds. When you see people you admire, who seem to be able to cope with their feelings and the difficulties in their lives, ask them what helps them through adversity.

Bernie: My occupation was both my wound and my teacher. I like people and I've always had the desire to help them, which is why I became a doctor. But I couldn't deal with the pain I felt when I was unable to heal everyone. For me, the initials *M.D.* came to mean "My Disease," and I had to find teachers to show me how to deal with my pain.

Be aware that in the hospital you may encounter people who don't know how to deal with their own emotions. You might even feel some of the staff pulling away from you. This could mean that you remind them of their own mortality—especially if you're the same age and sex. Or you might remind a doctor or nurse of a loved one whom they were unable to help, or even the person whose illness led them to choose a career in medicine or nursing.

If you sense that someone on the staff is uncomfortable with your illness, you can ask them about it and let them know that you can help them heal. Tell them that your disease isn't *their* disease. It may seem awkward to reach out to someone who's caring for you, but you can begin by asking, "How are you? How's your day going?" Or you can say, "Your job is a tough one—do you need a hug?" You can tell them what a difference they've made in your life. You might be surprised at how much a note of thanks or a symbolic gift can mean.

If you get the sense that your physician thinks *M.D.* stands for "My Discretion" or "Medical Deity," then it's definitely time to assert yourself. This is a person who wasn't adequately prepared by his or her training to care for patients. But by acting as a respant, you can break down the barrier he or she has put up and become your doctor's teacher. Begin by talking about how you're feeling about your treatment—not by complaining about and criticizing what your doctor is doing.

What to Pack

Healing objects. You may want to take some of the same items to the hospital that you'd take on vacation. Ask yourself, *What will help me relax and heal?* You can bring along pleasant aromas and room decorations that range from purely ornamental to personal and spiritual. You'll definitely want to bring items you've prepared specifically for your hospitalization—your meditation and visualization tapes, a tape or CD player, and your own personal healing objects.

You can create healing objects with your friends before you're hospitalized. What constitutes a healing object is entirely your decision, based upon your beliefs, experiences, aesthetics, and other preferences. People chose many types of healing objects— among them are mandalas, quilts, and mobiles. Some may already exist in your spiritual tradition—if not, you can create new objects and invest them with healing powers.

Look for objects that can easily be pinned on your hospital gown or hung on a wall, cubicle curtain, or ceiling. You'll want portable objects that you can carry to the hospital or rehabilitation center, and back to your home or wherever else you convalesce. Sometimes people combine efforts to create a healing object, such as sewing small squares together for a quilt. This can be done at your Vital Signs party, where your friends and family can give you blessings and other expressions of love and support as they contribute to your healing object.

Music. Music and healing sounds can serve as distractions from the noise and busyness of the hospital environment. Your music can help you feel more in control; when you listen to sounds of your choosing, you don't have to hear things that would otherwise be imposed on you. Music has been shown to be healing, soothing, comforting, relaxing, inspiring, sensual, and energizing. It will help you find harmony and rhythm wherever you are.

Music can help you connect with loved ones and with your past. Musical memory is one of the most resilient parts of our mind, and when other parts of the brain are impaired, musical memory may still be very much alive and ready to be tapped.

Yosaif: When my cousin was hospitalized in a semicomatose state with a severe brain injury, I brought my guitar to her bedside and sang to her. For a while she showed no sign of hearing the music. I kept moving from song to song, but still she didn't respond. Then I started singing an Israeli song she was familiar with and had an emotional connection to. With her eyes still closed, she slowly started moving her lips, and soon she was singing along in Hebrew. Remember: People can hear while asleep, in a coma, or under anesthesia.

Sometimes, the very moments we most need each other—moments of anguish, fear, and grief—are the times when it's most difficult to connect. Music can provide the connection. I know of a young woman who came back from surgery with the bad news that she had inoperable cancer. She and her mother were sitting together in silence, grieving separately, neither able to reach out to the other. Then they put on some music and looked into each others' eyes. Soon they were hugging and sobbing. Love filled the room and the healing process began for both mother and daughter.

When I was away from home for several weeks, acting as an advocate for my dad while he was recuperating from major cancer surgery, my friends brought me a homemade "Dr. Feelgood" tape with songs such as Bobby McFerrin's "Don't Worry, Be Happy." As a depleted caregiver, it certainly raised my spirits. You can make yourself a Dr. Feelgood tape, or ask a friend to make one for you. Producing the tape can be an opportunity for a great evening of brainstorming, listening to songs, and considering poems. These days, your musical choices are almost immediately available over the Internet. Since the world of Internet music is evolving quickly and there are legal copyright issues involved, I won't presume to advise you about how to find and record your favorite songs. However, if you know anyone younger than 15 years old, then you have an expert consultant.

The Internet and the innernet. Should you bring your computer to provide yourself Internet access? All we can say is, "Different strokes for different folks." For some, the World Wide Web may be the perfect bedside companion. It can connect you with people from all around the globe who care about you, and it can provide entertainment, music, news, medical information, bridge games, and endless information and interaction. While any of these Internet activities may be part of your healthy hospitalization, we don't recommend using your computer for anything you might label as "work."

Think carefully about what you need before you decide to remain connected to the Web. Your time in the hospital and recuperating at home are rare opportunities for you to have some serenity—this may be one of the best chances you'll ever have to experience your own inner life. Illness gives you a chance to take a break from multitasking and to focus on the single task of *being*. It's an opportunity to learn that others are capable of handling those responsibilities you thought only you could handle. When you're ill, you no longer need excuses for downtime—now it's handed to you as the silver lining of your illness.

Instead of spending hours on the Internet, you might want to take the rare opportunity to spend some time in the more serene place that Rabbi Zalman Schacter-Shalomi has dubbed the "innernet." There you may hear the silence that is the sweetest, most awe-inspiring, and sometimes the most frightening noise you'll ever hear—the sound of your soul.

Bedscapes®. These serene, comforting landscape pictures and tapes with the sounds of nature have helped many people heal.

> **Yosaif:** In the mid-1990s, I began providing hospitalized patients with landscapes that attach to cubicle curtains and audiotapes of natural sounds. In clinical studies, these Bedscapes® dramatically reduced the levels of stress and pain patients experienced. Today, Bedscapes® are found in hospices, nursing homes, intensive care units, and inpatient rooms in more than 50 hospitals. You can choose your own calming nature pictures and sounds, or find mine on-line at **www.bedscapes.com**.

Other items. You may want to bring along other objects, supplies, and props, such as flowers, religious symbols, stuffed animals, books, musical instruments, photos of your family and a bulletin board to display them, a clock, and special pillows and blankets.

If you have a pager, you can provide yourself with healing vibrations by setting it on "vibrate." Even if they're far away, your loved ones can send you good vibrations by calling your beeper whenever they're thinking healing, loving thoughts or sending prayers your way. (Check first to see if the hospital has any restrictions on the use of pagers.)

You can make yourself a "Loveline" out of clothespins and line. Attach this to your hospital cubicle curtain to hang objects that make you feel good—photos, cards, inspirational sayings, jokes, prayers, and affirmations. You can bring a treasure trove of healthy snacks for self-defensive eating—those times when you think the hospital meals aren't helping you heal.

Think about other practical items you might be glad to have with you: a mirror, hand and body lotions, a sleep mask, felt-tip pens and Magic Markers, masking tape or two-sided tape, blank index cards, large Post-it Notes (to make instant "thank-you" stickers to hand out to people), earplugs, or T-shirts with various messages ("Manager of Quality Assurance," "You Make a Difference," "VIP—Very Important Person"). You may also choose to bring an herbal pack that can be warmed in a microwave oven or cooled in a refrigerator. Such packs can be used to soothe any part of the body, but they're particularly comforting over the eyes.

Pack yourself a "Siegel Kit," including: a noisemaker you can use when you push the call button and get an hour of uninterrupted silence; a marker to write the appropriate message on your body when going to the O.R. for invasive, diagnostic tests; and a squirt gun to drench those who don't treat you with respect and honor your sacred space.

Photos of loved ones can provide comfort while you heal, but not many people know that a photo of *yourself* as an infant can work wonders, too. Everyone likes pictures of babies—even people who come into your room in a nasty mood are apt to ask, "Who's the cute kid?" Watch how their attitude changes when you answer, "Me!"

You may also want to display a photo of someone you admire, especially one who embodies the qualities you'll need on your current journey: courage, strength, humor, faith, equanimity, and so forth.

Although you can't bring your pets with you, if you're going to be hospitalized awhile, you might consider having them visit. If they aren't allowed in your room, you may be able to meet them in the lobby. Your family or team can have them bathed and checked by the vet before their visit. This is somewhat more permissible today, now that pet therapy is a recognized treatment.

Visitors are not an "item," but they're an important part of healing, so you should plan to provide yourself with some. But remember that respants make their own decisions: You can choose who you want to see. Ask them to be with you at the times you need them close by.

When children are hospitalized, love is their greatest healer—a hug or touch often does more good than a pill. So try to stay with your child throughout the day and night. If you can't be there, explain why you have to be away and be specific about when you'll be able to return. Leave tapes of your voice or the child's favorite music or nursery rhymes, and ask the nurse to play them.

> **Bernie:** Having a phone in the room doesn't mean you have to be at everyone's beck and call. You might decide to use the phone for a select group you know you'll want to talk to—spouse, children, co-workers. You may want to bring an answering machine or a phone that has caller identification so you can screen your calls (check whether your hospital has electronic specifications you need to comply with).
>
> You don't have to answer the phone, nor should you let it become an annoyance. In Buddhist countries, temple bells remind people to take a break from daily activities. We don't have temple bells here, we just have noise—but you can choose to let the ring or chirp of the phone be your call to mindfulness and spiritual calm. Let the telephone remind you to breathe peace and relax. Or you may turn off the ringer and let the answering machine provide you with white-room time. You don't have to answer the phone just because it rings—you aren't responsible for every problem in the universe.
>
> A woman once told me that she'd been contemplating suicide when the phone rang. "On the way to the phone," she said, "I realized that I don't have to commit suicide; I just have to stop answering the phone."

While you're preparing, don't forget to choose what attitude you want to bring to the hospital. Remember that a respant can make decisions about attitudes. Life is 10 percent what happens to you and 90 percent how you react to it, and happiness is an inside job—so if you're unhappy, make some changes. If you can, change the things that are disturbing you. If that's not possible, change your attitude toward whatever the problem is. Try following the advice Alcoholics Anonymous members give each other: Let go and let God [handle the difficult problems]. Or as Helen Keller said, "Keep your face to the sunshine and you cannot see the shadows." If you're making changes in your attitude, tell the people in your life what's happening and why so that they can understand and support you. *You can choose peace.*

Finally, what you *don't* bring with you may be as important as what you do bring. Be sure to leave behind that large sack filled with all of your worries, unfinished business, and imperfections. We all feel incomplete sometimes, and we're all still learning, but don't let your "incompleteness" stop you from doing everything you can to prepare for a healthy hospitalization. Remember:

- You're entitled to healing, no matter what your life experience has been.

- You're a divine child.

- You can learn to be master of your life's time.

- Something good will come of this.

- Every curse has its blessings.

Creating a Healing Sanctuary

If you have time to prepare and you want to do everything you can to ensure a healthy hospitalization, then you can create your own customized healing sanctuary. You might wonder why this is necessary—isn't the hospital itself supposed to be a healing sanctuary? In fact, modern hospitals are miracles of contradiction and paradox. Hospitals can provide you with sensory overload and sensory deprivation, social isolation and total lack of privacy—*all at the same time.* A miracle! But a miracle you don't need, and, with preparation, can avoid.

Think about the interesting model for portable healing environments that's been popping up everywhere, from airports to the streets of Manhattan: massage on-the-go. Right in the middle of the flurry of chaotic traffic—sights, sounds, odors, and dynamic human energy—the masseur or masseuse welcomes you to a sidewalk sanctuary. Here you can buy healing in ten-minute segments, usually at the cost of a dollar per minute. Most of us pass by these sidewalk healing vendors because we're too busy for that sort of thing. But the good news for you as you approach a hospital stay or at-home convalescence is that healing is now your first order of business. It's number one, two, and three on your list of priorities.

If a masseuse can create a healing sanctuary in the street, then you can certainly create one in a hospital bed. More and more patients are doing this, often on their own, without guidance from health-care professionals. You can start with the techniques our patients have shared with us. Your sanctuary, or psychic healing environment, must be custom-made for you if it's to have deep, healing meaning. The first step in creating your own sanctuary is developing images of what will help you heal. Begin by gathering paper, pencils, and crayons to make notes or draw pictures as you envision your healing sanctuary. You may want to draw images from your dreams, which are a rich source of ideas for healing sanctuaries.

The following exercise consists of questions aimed at helping you create a healing-friendly zone. Approach these questions as if they're a menu: You don't need to answer all the questions; you're choosing the ones that work for you. Don't let the exercise become work. Browse through the questions and start with the ones that speak to you.

Creating a Healing-Friendly Zone

Begin by reflecting on the kinds of things you enjoy having around—things that make you feel especially comforted and cared for. Think about the last time you were at home in bed with the flu and were feeling so sick that you simply had to let go of everything else and dedicate a few days solely to restoring yourself. What made you feel especially comforted? What kind of pillows, hand lotion, candles, incense, music, plants, and loved ones (human and other animals) did you want around? What was the lighting like? What made it easy to rest, sleep, and relax?

Some of the things you identify will be the types of things you can bring to the hospital; with others (your pets, for instance), you might need to do some extra negotiating and preparing. Make a preliminary list of things you and your friends can start gathering. Visitors will appreciate this—you give them a great gift when you provide them with specific ideas about how they can support you.

Everyone's healing sanctuary is unique, but a few qualities are common to most: safety, security, and comfort. You may already have a vision of what this means for you. Some people may say, "My bedside sanctuary is a soft cloud floating in warm air, and it's totally comforting and safe. When I'm in it, I feel love all around me, as if I'm being gently hugged," or "I feel like I'm lying in a hammock on a warm summer day, with gentle breezes blowing and birds singing."

Others who are more analytical may begin by looking at the definition of *sanctuary*. Dictionaries define sanctuaries as sacred or holy places, areas of asylum or protection, land where wildlife can breed and take safe refuge from hunters, and places that provide immunity from the law. The language is interesting. Notice the words *sacred, holy, immunity, refuge,* and *asylum.* The "land" is your bedside. Who or what are the hunters from whom you seek refuge? What are they hunting, and how can you protect yourself from them?

A sanctuary is a place where you—the human wildlife—feel safe and secure. What makes you feel that way? What makes you feel as if you're being cared for? What would help your healing? Sometimes we can discover positive things by first stating the negatives—such as qualities that would hinder or hamper your healing. It might help to ask, "What makes me feel as if I'm *not* being cared for?" "What *won't* help me heal?"

Think about a time when you felt especially serene and totally at ease. Where were you? What was especially pleasing about the setting? What did it feel like? What song immediately comes to mind when you think *serene, sanctuary, ease?* Sing that song to yourself—is there a message in it for you? How about a longer instrumental piece of music—perhaps classical or jazz? Might it be a wonderful soundtrack for your sanctuary?

What movie or play had a healing mood or theme, or a vivid scene that especially resonated with you? What character comes to mind? What might they bring to your sanctuary vision?

After you've thought about these questions, choose a half-dozen "quality" words to use as the foundation of your sanctuary. Next to each word, write one tangible object you could bring that embodies that quality. These objects can be sensory objects such as aromas, music, and textures.

As a centerpiece of your healing sanctuary, you or someone who cares about you can find or make a picture or symbol of your sanctuary to hang on your wall or cubicle curtain. From all the possible objects, select the one most likely to trigger and reinforce the feeling of being in a psychic-healing sanctuary. Then you and the rest of your team can start gathering other items and getting them ready for your hospital stay.

We're not suggesting that it will be easy to create an oasis amidst the constant turmoil of the hospital, but it can be done.

> **Yosaif:** My wife, Tsurah, knew that she had a true sanctuary when the nurses started spending more time in her room because they, too, needed a place that promoted healing.

> **Bernie:** I noticed something similar at my office. I'd often find my staff sitting in my consultation room, which was filled with healing symbols and objects.

If You Have No Time to Prepare

If you've had an accident or medical emergency that's left you with no time to prepare, you can still have a healthy hospitalization. Whether you're aware of it or not, your entire life has been preparation for healing. If you've learned from your difficulties and paid attention to the wisdom of others, then you're prepared for anything. If you haven't learned, and if you've never accepted the fact that you're mortal, then you may feel unprepared when you face serious difficulties. But it's never too late to begin healing.

If you're already in the hospital—and you arrived without any preparation, Vital Signs, healing objects, or group of friends to help you—know that you can still start to put together a healing team, make drawings, begin guided visualizations, and create a healing sanctuary. Remember, your preparation doesn't have to be perfect. You don't have to do everything, and you're not being graded. This isn't about perfection; it's about being a survivor, acting responsibly, and participating in the process of healing. Just begin by being a respant, and do what you can to get on a healing path. In the next chapter, we'll focus on the hospital environment and talk about ways you can adapt it so that it supports your efforts to heal.

᠎ﾞﾞ

CHAPTER 4

Crossing the Threshold:
How to Behave Like a
Respant in the Hospital

You can't experience true healing without love, but unfortunately, you may encounter the opposite of love in the hospital. If that statement confuses you, remember that the opposite of love isn't hate or fear—it's indifference. You can make preparations as a respant before your hospitalization, but once you cross the threshold, you'll have to *continue* behaving respantly if you want people to pay attention to your needs and not just your diagnosis.

Remember why you didn't prepare yourself to be a "good patient": The people identified as such by nurses are the ones who die the fastest. Nice patients undergo medical treatment and operations someone else has prescribed for them, and they bear annoyance, pain, and suffering without getting angry or complaining. They manage to give the appearance of being unruffled and self-composed. We're taught to think that those are good traits, and that they make it easier for medical personnel to care for you, but remaining nonchalant about receiving the wrong treatment can kill you.

When we say that you need to be empowered to get the attention you deserve, we're not suggesting that you think of yourself as an animal trainer cracking a whip. Empowerment doesn't mean bullying people or creating adversaries. When you're truly empowered, you know that love is always the weapon of choice.

Bernie: Years ago, when airline personnel would argue with me over the size of my carry-on luggage, I used to show them that I could fit my bag into the measuring frame. I was always able to demonstrate that I was right, but I never once won the argument this way.

One day, as I was preparing to board, I realized that I needed to practice what I preached, and that meant changing tactics. Instead of self-righteously heading for the measuring rack, I looked at the attendant with empathy and said, "I need your love." She let me board and moved on to argue with the person behind me.

When you encounter indifference in the hospital, you don't have to be nasty or argumentative, unpleasant or haughty. You can get people's attention by asking for it directly, the way Bernie asked the flight attendant for her love. Your goal is to help others see you as an individual with needs.

Behaving Like a Respant in the Hospital

Being empowered means knowing—or finding out—what you're getting into. You wouldn't sign a blank contract outside the hospital, so don't sign one inside, either. Before you give someone permission to do surgery or other medical procedures, make sure you know all the details. For example, consenting to an appendectomy means agreeing to anesthesia, too. So ask detailed questions about possible side effects, likely complications, and hoped-for benefits. Then allow yourself some time to think about what you've been told. If the staff gives you information that makes you fearful immediately before your procedure, cancel it and have it done another day, after you've had time to process everything.

Frightened patients are more likely to experience cardiac arrest in the operating room—you can literally be scared to death.

You may think that reading your paperwork is unnecessary because the person asking you to sign probably knows what the forms mean, but *you* need to know, too. Look over every form carefully; signing a permission slip for an operation opens you up to many risks.

> **Bernie:** I once had a man show up in the operating room who had signed an operative permit giving me permission to perform a hysterectomy. The man was already sedated, so I had to postpone surgery because we couldn't ask him to sign the proper permit while he was under the effect of drugs. This wouldn't have happened if, when he was given the forms to read the night before, he had understood the importance of really reading them.

Unless you're involved in a disastrous emergency, you'll usually have enough time to ask everyone to step back and give you some time to discuss things with your surgeon, person-to-person. This obviously doesn't apply if you're close to death or unable to communicate—in that case your family will want to move ahead with a physician they know, or one whom your family doctor trusts.

Question authority. You may be hesitant to question the medical staff, especially those physicians who think *M.D.* means "Medical Deity." But a respant knows that it's always appropriate to question authority. Don't learn the hard way that the people in charge of your care can make mistakes. You have every right—and as a respant you have the *responsibility*—to inquire about the reputation of the hospital and the qualifications of the people caring for you.

Ask your doctor if he or she is board certified or has ever been professionally disciplined or lost hospital privileges. You can ask, "How experienced are you in treating my condition?" "How have your patients done compared with other patient groups?" "What outcome, complications, and risks should I be prepared for if I accept your treatment suggestions—and if I choose not to?" Feel free to inquire about how often a procedure is performed at the hospital, and ask to talk to other patients who have the same diagnosis and were offered the same treatment. Find out about their experiences with the hospital staff and prescribed regimen.

Again, this is not adversarial. When you ask these questions, let your medical or surgical team know that this isn't directed at them because of any negative feelings, threats, or fears. You're asking because you sincerely want to be an empowered member of your own treatment team, and you can't say yes to their suggested therapy if you have unanswered questions.

Intuition is a tool that can help you question authority and make your own decisions. Use your intuition to maintain a sense of what's right for you. If you're waiting for a test and the procedure is delayed, you can get up and leave—if that feels right for you. But think about your feelings first: Does it really feel right to leave, or are you just annoyed by the delay? During your wait you might meet someone whose advice or recommendation saves your life.

Be a scurvy elephant. If you aren't sure how to interact with people in the hospital, you can always remember the scurvy elephant story a cancer patient once told Bernie. Her son came home from school one day and said that his teacher had called him a "scurvy elephant." Naturally, the woman went to the school the next day to find out what could have prompted such a comment. The teacher laughed and replied, "You have a bright son who's always speaking up—I said he's sometimes a *disturbing element.*" Later, when the mother was hospitalized for cancer treatment, she realized that she needed to become a "scurvy elephant" to get the treatment she needed.

The Siegel Kit you packed in Chapter 3 will help you become a scurvy elephant in the hospital. When you push the call button and an hour passes with no response, use your noisemaker. Get out your Magic Marker and write on your body before you go in for surgery or invasive diagnostic tests. And use the squirt gun on those who don't treat you with respect.

Some of the other items you packed will be useful now. Get out your special gown or clothing embroidered with V.I.P.— which stands for "Very Important *Person*," not *"Patient."* Unpack the photographs and items from home that will help you heal and give you a sense of security. Set up your Bedscape. Use your music, aromas, and guided-imagery tapes to create your healing environment. Unpack your childlike sense of humor, and put the signs you've created on your door to let hospital staff and visitors know how they can help you.

Check to see if you're on a healing path. While you're convalescing, you can make a conscious choice to follow a healing path. Psychiatrist George Solomon developed a set of questions to identify people who are likely to be long-term survivors, and we touched on some of these survival traits in Chapter 1 when we discussed empowerment. It's always the right time to ask yourself Dr. Solomon's questions about how you're living, but it's especially important that you take this inventory when you're facing illness. So read through the questions, and answer them as you go. You may also benefit from meditating, praying, and visualizing on them. To see if you're on a healing path, ask yourself:

- *Do I have a sense of meaning in my work, daily activities, family life, and relationships?* Make a conscious decision about how you'll contribute love and serve others. This is your choice—don't look to anyone else to decide this for you.

- *Am I able to express anger appropriately in defense of myself?* If you're not treated with respect, speak up or use your squirt gun. If you internalize anger, you're more likely to become sick, and you'll end up full of resentment and hate, which will hurt you and those around you.

- *Am I able to ask friends and family for support when I'm feeling lonely or troubled?* Being polite isn't the same thing as being a doormat. You need to share your pain and let others help you to heal. If you deny your pain to make their lives easier, then you're hurting yourself.

- *Am I able to ask friends and family for favors when I need them?* Don't be afraid to ask for favors. Let your family and friends know that you don't mean to impose on them—you need help, but they're free to say no if they can't provide what you want or need.

- *Am I able to say no to someone who asks for a favor if I can't do it or don't feel like doing it?* This is the most important question for you and for everyone on your team. The key is doing what feels right for you and for others. Gifts given out of love benefit both the giver and the receiver, but gifts given out of guilt damage relationships. To be healthy, you need to feel free to say no.

- *Do I engage in health-related behaviors based on my own self-defined needs instead of someone else's prescriptions or ideas?* Don't let others tell you what pain to experience or what treatments to undergo in an effort to avoid dying. When you make the decisions about your care, you reduce the number and severity of side effects you'll experience. Life is a labor pain, but you choose what pain you're willing to experience to give birth to yourself.

- *Do I have enough play in my life?* When you're doing something that makes you lose track of time, you're in the state that's healthiest for your mind and body.

- *Do I find myself depressed for long periods, during which time I feel hopeless about changing the conditions that cause me to be depressed?* Don't get depressed about being depressed! As we explained in Chapter 1, you can have a productive depression if you use your pain and let your feelings redirect you—just as you let hunger direct you to seek food.

- *Am I dutifully filling a prescribed role in my life (wife, nice guy, parent) to the detriment of my own needs?* If you live a role, your life may end when the need for that part approaches an end. Instead of limiting yourself to one function, find your unique, authentic self—and live that life.

If you answered yes to the first seven questions and no to the last two, then you're already on a healing path. If those aren't your answers, then you know where you have work to do.

Making the "Right" Choices

We've talked about the importance of being empowered, and we've given you tips on how to reach that state. But you may have noticed that we haven't said a lot about the specific decisions you'll make when you're empowered. That's because we don't know what decisions are right for you; empowerment isn't a one-size-fits-all proposition. What's right for one person may be wrong for someone else—that's what makes human beings such an interesting species.

It's important that you appreciate and respect your own coping style. Two empowered people can make entirely different decisions about the details of their hospitalization and treatment—anesthesiologists have known this for a long time. Some people want to be so heavily sedated that when they're roused they can't believe they've already been operated on. Others want to be as close to awake as possible so that they know everything that's going on, and there are those who choose to avoid sedating drugs entirely, opting to use acupuncture or hypnosis. The people who want to be unconscious think you'd have to be crazy to want to be awake, while the people who choose acupuncture wouldn't do it any other way because they don't want to have to recover from both the surgery and the anesthesia.

People may also have different feelings about surgery, chemotherapy, radiation, exercise, and maintaining a healthy diet. Some may see a particular therapy as a blessing, whereas others can't help but view it as a mutilation or burden. Individuals who regard their treatment as a gift will have fewer side effects, so in one sense they have a better perspective. But those who know they can't manage such a positive view should make choices based on what they feel, not on what someone else tells them to do.

In some cases, patients want their doctors to act like shamans and perform "magic" for them. They don't want any active involvement themselves, and they don't want any explanations or details. They simply put their faith in the doctor and hope for the best. Many studies have shown that this isn't the healthiest approach, but they have the right to choose that kind of care if that's what they want.

You, on the other hand, may prefer a much more active role. As you think about healing and gather information, you may decide to be your own primary caregiver. You can research the medical approaches that are available, choose the providers you feel best about, and direct your own treatment. If this is your usual style, you may find that right now, because of your illness, your mind-set or energy level doesn't allow you to be quite as involved and assertive as you normally are. You may need someone else on your team to be available as your advocate until you can move back into the driver's seat.

So which course is right: the more passive or more active? The answer is both—depending on who you are and what your immediate situation is. You can choose a more hands-off approach and still be a respant—if that's the right choice for you at this moment.

However, be aware that you may change your strategy as your situation changes, or as your feelings about yourself, your illness, and your healing evolve. You may want to enhance and transform your style in response to your current illness, but don't let yourself be coerced into making choices that feel wrong. Remember, you're both the artist *and* the work of art.

Being empowered means trusting your own judgment about what feels best for you, and not worrying about what you *think* should feel best. We don't want you to feel guilty about any choices you make, because you're the only one in your situation right now. Our guide to empowered behavior is designed to be useful for any type of patient, because we offer many coaching tips but only one prescription: *Make choices that feel right for you.*

Getting Oriented

The transition from ordinary "civilian" life to hospital life can be one of the most abrupt changes you'll ever have to make, especially if you're admitted in an emergency situation. To feel a sense of control and self-sufficiency, it helps to know where you are and how you got there. It's not enough to be told, "You're now in a major teaching hospital associated with an outstanding medical school"—you need a visceral understanding of where the hospital is in relation to the world that's familiar to you. (If you're reading this because someone you love is a patient, don't underestimate how much good you can do by helping to provide a basic orientation. You're helping your loved one heal when you help him or her get acclimated after admission, or on returning from the recovery room after surgery.)

If you arrived in an ambulance or under other emergency circumstances, you'll not only need to get a sense of where you are within the hospital, you'll also need to find out what hospital you're in and what kind of reputation it has. Of course if you came in on your own steam, you already have a sense of where the hospital is in relation to where you live, but you may not have a clear picture of where your room is in relation to the nurses' station, lobby, and your ultimate destination—the exit, which in most hospitals is the front door. If you're ambulatory, take a few minutes to figure all this out. If you're bedridden, have someone help you, but take your time and don't expend too much energy. Healing is more important than mapping the hospital's geography. You can always ask the world's most frequently asked question when you need to: "Where's the bathroom?"

It can be confusing, even dizzying, to see all the different people who come in and out of your room. Some of these individuals are there to perform different tasks, and some perform the same task, but on different shifts or different days of the week. Find out who all these people are and let them know who you are. Ask how they can help you to heal. Show them that they're not just faceless people to you by asking about them, and caring about them as people. That will help them to see you for who you are—a person—and not a disease or condition.

Here's an orientation list to help you demystify your hospital experience. If you or your advocate gathers this information early in your stay, you'll feel grounded and confident that your healing needs will be met. As with all of our lists, don't feel responsible for accomplishing every item. These are suggestions we offer for your benefit. Do the ones that feel right for you and ignore the rest.

- Learn who's responsible for your care.

- Ask a loved one to begin a list of "Hospital-speak"—words that hospital staff use that ordinary mortals don't understand (or understand differently). Then periodically ask your nurse or doctor to translate them for you.

- Ask your attending nurse to help you draw a diagram of the professional caregivers attending to you. Begin this drawing with yourself in the center, and use circles to represent your attending physician, primary nurses, specialists, and assigned residents (if any). Use this diagram as a reference when a staff member comes to visit you at your bedside.

- Ask about the general daily rhythm of hospital life around you. On what schedule can you expect major things to be done for you or to you?

- Ask about any major treatment changes that are planned for the day—this is a task you'll need to repeat each day.

- Learn the hospital geography—this is especially important if you're ambulatory, but if you're not, it's still important information for your family. Where is the family lounge, cafeteria, library, chapel or meditation room, room with computers or Internet access, gift shop, outside healing garden, and so forth?

Your Healing Team in the Hospital

Too often the hospital experience is one of scarcity—scarcity of love, soothing touch, humor, variety, space, perspective, fresh air, and staff. But your stay can be different. You can open the gates to let love flow in, and provide yourself with abundant health care by developing your own healing team.

If you were able to read Chapter 3 before becoming a patient, you may have already put together a team that includes you, your family, visitors, health-care professionals, and whatever higher power or spiritual force you feel a connection to. But don't forget that in the hospital, you'll encounter many people whom you'll want to add to your team, and most will be happy to join you.

Health-care workers get their deepest satisfaction from helping people. Sadly, they often find that much of their day is consumed with depersonalizing busywork that has little to do with healing. They'd really rather be helping patients whenever they can, so by forming a team that includes the hospital staff, you become their ally. Because you have your own support group, you're not just another patient who's dependent on the staff for all your needs. Certainly you'll have some requests and demands for them, but you'll be making them from the perspective of a fellow team member who's helping move the ball toward the goal line.

As we said in Chapter 3, when you establish a healing team, sit down with the members and outline what you expect from them. If anyone is unwilling or unable to perform what you ask, find someone else to do it. With your family and your physician, you may want to write out or discuss an agreement with guidelines for all of you to follow. You don't need a formal written contract with the hospital staff, and you don't necessarily need to discuss team membership, but you *do* need a sense that you all have a mutual agreement to focus on your healing.

Believe it or not, most hospitals already have an unstated, de facto contract with their patients. It goes something like this: *You come here with proper insurance coverage, and we'll provide our medical technology and services to fix what's wrong with you. We'll repair you and send you home.* It's pretty much like bringing your car in for some bodywork and letting the guys at the shop do what they know how to do best. In this case, you can't drop off your body, so you have to stick around while the work is being done. During your stay, you're not expected to make demands any more than your car would.

There's a problem with that contract, because you're bringing in a lot more than your body—more than even your "condition" or, as it's called in Hospital-speak, your D.R.G. (**d**iagnostic **r**elated **g**roup). Your body, at its deepest cellular level, contains the smart technology that allows it to be self-correcting and self-healing—if you give it the right circumstances in which to operate. You're different from your car—you need a shop that pays attention to your body, mind, and spirit—so you need a contract different from the one you have with your mechanic.

The *Help Me to Heal* contract aims at providing you with maximum healing and comfort. It's a given that you expect to be able to choose from the best technology the hospital has to offer. But for you to gain the maximum benefit from that technology, your own inner environment must be allowed to do what it was designed to do—help you to heal. For that, you need your bedside zone to become your healing sanctuary, you need to be able to be as active as you want to be in choosing your treatment, and your healing team needs to be empowered to help you make decisions. Your contract with the hospital should acknowledge that you have all these human needs.

One final note on your contract with your team: Your body is a gift with which you love, serve others, and experience life. The contract you make with your team should make it clear that when your body has lost its ability to serve and you're tired and sore, you can choose to leave. This doesn't make you a failure. You're human, and your death is inevitable—but you have some choice over the timing.

Don't be afraid to share your feelings about death with your team. Some of the members may have difficulty with the thought of your death, but that shouldn't mean that you have to suffer excessively, trying to avoid dying for their sake. Nor should you have to die alone to relieve team members of their distress. A respant gets to decide when hospice care is in order. We've been saying that healing is about living in peace, but it's also about dying in peace. Death is not a failure.

Bernie: We'd like you to be able to die laughing. This is possible if you have several important needs fulfilled. First, you need to know that you've accomplished what you were sent here to accomplish, and that love is immortal and serves as the bridge between the land of the living and the dead. The second thing you need is to hear your family tell stories about your life. When they get going, you can die as my father did, smiling and laughing at the stories my mother was telling about their first dates.

When the moment is right for you, the transition out of this life will be a spiritual experience and your next form of therapy. I see this in many people's drawings, where ascending purple kites or balloons symbolize a heavenly journey. One day I asked my 90-year-old father-in-law, who was quadriplegic from a fall, if he had any insight about aging successfully. He said, "Fall on something soft." The next day he said, "Well, that doesn't always work. They stood me up in therapy, and I fell over on my wife and broke her leg. My advice is: Just fall up." I laughed, but not long after, he showed me what the final healing can be like. One night he refused his vitamins and dinner, and then died. It seemed that he really did just fall up, because he became dreamless, unalive, and perfect.

I feel I can guarantee you that it's possible to fall up and that consciousness lives on. That's not really the point of this book, but it's worth noting that people are making fascinating discoveries about memories stored in transplanted organs, near-death experiences, and past-life regressions. If you want to learn more about these subjects, there are many resource books available to help you. Here we're only going to ask you to open your mind and accept that life is a mystery. If you can experience life as a mystery, you'll encounter the faith that heals. In the words of T. S. Eliot: "So the darkness shall be the light, and the stillness the dancing."

As the leader of your own healing team, you're also in charge of Quality Assurance. In this role, your job is to ensure that you get what you need, when you need it. You're in charge of being vigilant about what procedures are done to you, what medications are brought, and what foods are served. It might be a good idea to keep the names and phone numbers of some key hospital staff at your bedside. We suggest that you know how to contact the director of patient representation, the medical director, the director of nursing, the director of quality, and the director of marketing or public relations. Of course we hope you never have to use any of these numbers, but if you aren't getting satisfactory care, you may want to inform someone on this list that you're not getting the healing attention you need. Let them know that your next step will be to call the Joint Commission on Accreditation of Healthcare Organizations (JCAHO) (complaint hot line: 800-994-6610, or **complaint@jcaho.org**), your state's department of health hot line, or a reporter for your local television station.

Knowing Your Rights

Every hospital is required by law and by the JCAHO guidelines to post a copy of a patient's bill of rights. You and your advocates need to be familiar with your rights and know how to exercise them.

Generally, you have the right to: be treated with respect, know the names and functions of all staff attending to you, have access to all the information you need to make proper medical choices, and have your choices respected and complied with.

Recently, patients' bills of rights have been amended to include the right to adequate pain relief, which means having your pain assessed and addressed in a way that makes you comfortable. Illness and convalescence are not times to be stoic and suffer—that's not survival behavior. Living with unnecessary pain may inhibit your sleep, which is vital to your healing.

The change in attitudes toward pain management grew out of studies showing that most physicians are inadequately trained in diagnosing and treating pain, and that it's widely undertreated.

This is the one area where physicians undermedicate their patients, usually in the mistaken belief that pain medications will be addictive. In fact, there are pain-management regimens that mitigate the risk of addiction, and special methods are available for treating patients with histories of substance abuse.

There has been other progress recently in the area of pain management. Hospitals are implementing medical and nursing protocols to ensure that patients receive adequate relief, and at the same time, they're accelerating their in-service training in pain management to fill the gap in medical and nursing education. Many health-care professionals are beginning to view pain as a "fifth vital sign" that requires continual assessment and treatment. One simple scheme allows patients to rate their discomfort on a one-to-ten scale—the staff then treats the pain the individual is feeling, rather than the pain they think the patient should experience with a particular procedure or affliction.

One last issue should be highlighted: You have a right to have your cultural, religious, and/or spiritual practices respected. You may not be allowed to kill a chicken in your room, but you have a right to be served a healthy alternative to pork if you're a Muslim, Jew, or Seventh-day Adventist. If you're a Hindu, you're entitled to a beef substitute. These are basic human rights, and continuing your cultural practices and maintaining your spiritual traditions are vital to your healing.

The Odd Coupling: Becoming Foxhole Buddies

If we need to be in the hospital, most of us would prefer to be in a private room. It may be well worth dipping into your savings (if you're lucky enough to have some) to pay a few hundred extra dollars for the peace and quiet you need at this particularly vulnerable moment in your life. A private room doesn't free you from the twin hospital paradoxes—sensory deprivation combined with sensory overload, and social isolation coupled with total lack of privacy—but it does allow you more freedom to make your space complement your healing.

Often, the best available accommodation is a semiprivate room. These rooms often come with a roommate, and the matching process is generally random—but a little company might turn out to be just what you need. We know of many instances where someone's roommate turned out to be a real blessing. You may think that this is one of those times when you're going to have to just make the best of a bad situation, but you might be surprised by how much healing potential there is in forced cohabitation. Instead of gritting your teeth and trying to ignore your roommate, you might want to open up to your new "foxhole buddy" and seek goodness in your relationship.

Yosaif: I have two hospital roommate experiences that illustrate the range of possibilities. The first took place shortly after I arrived at a hospital in New York City for an operation on a parotid gland tumor. At first I couldn't believe what they'd done to me: They put me in a room with a dying man who was moaning. The moaning was bad enough, but worse were all the other respiratory sounds—pained breathing, wheezing, and mucus being brought up and spat out.

When I'd settled in, Sammy and I exchanged brief introductory formalities. He was a family man and a retired longshoreman from the piers of the Red Hook section of Brooklyn—Marlon Brando's *On the Waterfront* territory. We fell into a conversational groove, and it was easy, neither terribly engaging nor terribly demanding. I forget what we talked about, but I remember that as we talked I relaxed, and stopped wishing that I wasn't sharing a space with Sammy. Despite our very different life paths, we'd both found our way to Dr. Conley, a world-renowned cancer surgeon, and to this particular hospital room where we were in the process of evolving from involuntary room-mates to foxhole buddies.

The night before my surgery, I had a high fever. For some reason, the nurses didn't seem to pay any attention to the fever and the fact that I was freezing and shudder-ing in my hospital bed. So Sammy became my advocate, demanding that they bring me extra blankets and tend to my chills.

The morning of my surgery, Sammy kept up a con-stant chatter—of the most affirming kind. "Kid, the oper-ation's a piece of cake. That Dr. Conley's done 2,000 of these—he's even invented the ways to deal with any prob-lems that might come up. You'll be fine."

I was, and when I got back from the postsurgical recovery area, there was Sammy, welcoming me back to our room. So the dying longshoreman I hadn't wanted to meet ended up being my mentor and teacher. I came away from that experience convinced that we have healing angels all around us—we just need to slow down, notice them, and open ourselves to their gifts.

My father, on the other hand, wasn't so lucky. After undergoing a 16-hour, two-team operation and spending several days in the Medical Intensive Care Unit (MICU), he was taken to a semiprivate room. His roommate was very big, very angry, very loud, and very unhappy to see us.

My dad had been courageous in deciding to have the surgery and facing all the challenges in the days he was preparing for it. Now, postoperative, he was weak and shaken. He had tubes going in and out of his nose and mouth, and he could no longer speak because his larynx had been removed. His temperament was intense, but his delicate sensibilities were intact. I was sure he would thrive if he could only listen to Brahms, do *The New York Times* cross-word puzzle (in ink!), and use his CPA expertise to advise the nurses how to handle their income-tax problems. But it was difficult to establish the tone my father needed in a room with this hulking and belligerent roommate. Fortunately, the angry man checked out after 24 hours, which was 24 hours too late as far as we were concerned.

While your roommate may be dauntingly incompatible with you, he or she may also help you. Simply having another person in the room may provide safety and security, and you may find that it's a relief to both of you to unburden yourselves in conversation. You might find yourself telling your roommate things that you wouldn't be comfortable discussing with the people closest to you—how you're *really* doing, what you're afraid of, what's working in your life that you can't wait to get back to, and what needs fixing. One of the most important things you and your roommate can do is serve as nonjudgmental witnesses for each other.

At times, roommates also become empowering advocates for one another, the way Sammy was. You may find yourself sharing insights into the medical system and ideas about how to deal with your conditions or certain members of the hospital staff. Sometimes roommates even make healing pacts with each other— vowing to recover and meet outside in the civilian world to do something fun together.

When you're getting to know your roommate, remember that everyone is wounded and there are reasons why people behave as they do. Don't be afraid to ask questions, and when you have a complaint, express how you feel. If you begin the discussion by saying, "You're a problem," you may not have a productive conversation. But if you say, "*I'm* having a problem," then you can expect the kind of dialogue that promotes healing. You can find the balance you both need if you're explicit about what you will and will not do in the room; and when, how often, and how. Don't forget to discuss the behavior of your visitors. Some of the things you might want to reach agreement about are:

- noise of all types, including voices, television, music, and telephone sounds;

- intrusions and respect for each other's space; and

- aromas—one person's delight can drive another to distraction, as smell is one of the most powerful and primitive senses.

You may want to agree on a way to signal each other when noise is disturbing, or one of you wants to be alone. Be aware that you may need to change your agreement as your convalescence proceeds and your (or your roommate's) needs change.

After considering all this, you may still want to dig into your savings and pay for a private room. But if you choose to have a roommate, you may find that this transient relationship with a stranger turns out to be one of the most rewarding relationships you'll have in your life. It may even help you to heal.

Remember that the key is *communication;* your healing may depend on your willingness and ability to tell people what you need. In the next chapter, we'll show you one of the best ways to make your unique needs known to roommates, medical staff, family, and anyone else you encounter while you're in the hospital.

జు

CHAPTER 5

Creating Vital Signs

Vital Signs can be posted by you and your loved ones on your door or cubicle curtain to let everyone know what you need and how they can help you heal. They can be used in a hospital, assisted-living facility, nursing home, or any other environment in which you're convalescing (including your own home!). The signs are an easy way to focus everyone's attention on your needs at a time when you want to conserve your energy—and don't want to have to do a lot of explaining and reminding.

Here are some examples of Vital Signs we've seen patients use over the years:

- Healing in progress. . . . Please come back in 15 minutes.

- Trying to rest; please keep your voices down. Thank you.

- Being present here is the best gift you can give me.

- Welcome to Wellsville!

These really are Vital Signs in the sense that they're vitally important to your healing. Of course, the term also refers to the other "vital signs" that play such a central role in hospital life: your pulse, blood pressure, temperature, and respiratory rate (and, as we mentioned in the previous chapter, some hospitals have recently begun monitoring a fifth vital sign—pain). The staff members at health-care facilities pay very close attention to these signs in order to detect changes in your condition, but we want the people caring for you to pay as much attention to your need for rest, privacy, and love as they pay to your pulse and temperature.

You don't need a lot of training to create Vital Signs; you just need to remember that you deserve to be cared for with love and respect. That isn't something you earn—it's a right that you're born with. If you're skeptical about this, turn to the "Entitlement Learner's Permit" in Part III, and refer back to it whenever you begin to doubt that you're worthy of such treatment. Don't let your past experiences keep you from expressing your needs.

Do you feel uncomfortable telling people how they can help you? Do you wonder whether you have the right to hang up signs in a hospital? This may come as a surprise to you, but the hospital bed you're in right now "belongs" to you for as long as you occupy it. So does your portion of the room. A hospital room is no different than a hotel room—it's yours as long as you pay for it. You have as much right to hang up signs in it as you do in a hotel room.

In most cases, you also have the right to leave the hospital by simply signing out, the same as you would at a hotel. You might be told that you're leaving "against medical advice," but nonetheless, it's your prerogative. It's your life, your illness, and your choice. We're not advocating that you check out of the hospital before you're ready or against your doctor's orders; we're just acknowledging that you have the right to choose whether to stay, go home, or move to another facility. We want you to remember that you're not a prisoner—you *can* leave. When you know you have that option, you'll be more apt to insist on receiving intensive caring 24/7 for as long as you choose to stay.

You're entitled to 'round-the-clock care if you need it, but you obviously can't expect any one person to be on duty all of the time. Nobody works 24-hour shifts, except interns and residents, and that kind of schedule isn't healthy for them (but that's another story). Except for residents, everybody goes off duty regularly so that they can take care of themselves.

But oddly enough, people expect patients to be on duty all the time. While you're hospitalized, the staff will assume that you're available at all hours of the day and night for the procedures and routines involved in your care. This usually includes a lot of people coming in and going out of your room, and the nurses and doctors are apt to assume that you'll adapt to their schedules and undergo testing and treatment at their discretion. You'll be expected to remain stationary and passive—the traditional, submissive, suffering patient—always "on." It may never occur to anyone that you need a moment of privacy or control over your space and time, so it's your job as a respant, armed with Vital Signs, to turn the *on* around and say *no*.

It may surprise you that you can say no, or that you can insist on some privacy. "Privacy? In a hospital? You must be kidding, right? Patients can't have privacy, can they?" you may ask. Yet the people who study wellness will tell you that you need some control over your mind, body, and spirit. This need doesn't evaporate when you become a patient—if anything, it becomes more crucial. In the best of circumstances, you still can't control everything, but your everyday routine may afford you a sense of order in the details of your life. When you're forced to live by someone else's schedule, you lose this regularity, and it's normal to feel a great deal of stress. If you're always on call, your spirit and immune system will suffer. Stress, spiritual malaise, a suppressed ability to fight disease—that's a prescription for illness, not healing.

If you want to heal, try establishing some routines in your new environment. Taking a 15-minute "serenity break" every 24 hours is a good start, although we recommend doing this every 4 to 6 hours. These short respites pay huge dividends in how you feel, and they simultaneously remind your caregivers that you're a lot more than a "patient." You're a human being with a soul, imagination, feelings, and aspirations. You can emphasize who you are by doing what owners of private roads do to maintain their ownership rights—periodically, they close off the road to assert their right of control over it. You can close off your private sanctuary for 15 minutes at least once a day to establish ownership over yourself, and to give yourself time that you can call serenity time, Sabbath or white-room time, feeling-free time, gone-fishin' time, or just plain *life* time.

Taking control is a three-step process:

1. **Select or create the necessary signs.** If you made signs at a prehospitalization Vital Signs party, you may already have what you need. If not, you and your team can make the signs you need now.

2. **Negotiate with the staff.** The nurses can help you identify the best times of the day for taking your breaks. Ask them about their schedules and the schedules of other staff: doctors, housekeeping staff, technicians, and food-service workers. The doctors' schedules may seem unpredictable, but there are patterns—and the nurses know them.

3. **Post your Vital Signs.** Hang your chosen signs on your door or cubicle curtain to let everyone know your intentions, and then close the door or curtain at the appropriate time.

Vital Signs are meant to help you establish your sacred time and space. After your first time going through the three step process—selecting or creating, negotiating, and posting—you may feel more confident and entitled to turn your bedside environment into your own healing zone. Now you're ready to dream up and broadcast other messages that will help you build your healing sanctuary, turn visits into healing encounters, and invite people to join your healing team.

Soon you'll be thinking of all sorts of new ways to use Vital Signs. You can spell out the qualities you want people to bring into your space, such as love, humor, honesty, equanimity, or ease. Maybe you'll have some signs focusing on qualities you want to keep *out* of your space—such as fear, worry, guilt, and pretense. You may want to post signs asking your roommate's visitors to speak softly or keep the volume on the television down—but talk this over with your roommate first, and present it as a need, not as a criticism.

It's also a good idea to post messages directed toward your health-care professionals: reminders that you're a lot more than a "patient," expressions of gratitude to people who are part of your healing team, and invitations for others to help you to heal.

Keep these ideas in mind while you're composing Vital Signs:

- You want to promote your three *Help Me to Heal* goals (creating a healing sanctuary, healing visits, and a healing team).

- You want to put out healing energy and get that energy circulating around you.

- Your bywords are *love* and *loving*.

- Your signs are invitations or invocations: For example, "It will help me to heal if you would . . . [fill in the blank]." This is more likely to be effective than posting biblical injunctions and threatening fire and brimstone to those who don't comply.

- You want to avoid inappropriate anger, and you don't want to induce guilt, blame, or shame.

More Examples of Vital Signs

Here are some more Vital Signs that other patients have created and posted:

- Love is the only language spoken here. (Or "Aquí se habla amor.")

- I invite you to leave your worries on the doorstep.

- All we need is love.

- No need to worry—I've already delegated worrying to somebody else!

- Let's be silent for the first minute of our visit.

- My insurance company and I see eye-to-eye: We both want me out of here as quickly as possible!

- How may I help you?

- How will what you're about to do help me to heal?

- When in doubt, try the loving way.

- Since we all know that life has a 100% mortality rate, let's not sweat the small stuff.

- Bernie Siegel told me to do this!

- Unless otherwise indicated, I'm not hard of hearing—
  so please speak to me in a normal tone of voice.

- Unless I request it, please only keep the indirect (upward)
  light on. Thank you. [**Note:** This one is for posting above
  the switch for the overhead fluorescent light.]

- I'm my primary Quality Assurance Manager—
  please help me do my job.

- You make a difference!

- The beautiful baby in the accompanying photo is me.

- $5 fee for all visits and examinations.

While you're creating Vital Signs, remember that your purpose
is holy, but the signs themselves are not. Be charitable and forgiving with people when they first experience your signs. Some people might joke about them while they try their best to make sense
of what you're up to. Believe it or not, the signs that cause the
most initial discomfort for the staff are the ones that express gratitude to them.

That's all there is to Vital Signs. It may take a few tries before
they work smoothly, so just rehearse and practice and ask for constructive criticism and ideas. People aren't used to the idea of
patients going off duty to heal—but you can help them get used to
it. You can be a pioneer in the Vital Signs movement. When
patients in hospital beds all over the world start hanging up signs
and taking sacred time for themselves, we'll know that a profound
shift is taking place and that health care is becoming "healing care."

Until that happens, you can use your Vital Signs to provide
yourself with healing moments of serenity, affection, humor, control, ease, and honesty. Your experience with Vital Signs will whet

your appetite and spur you to look for more ways to provide yourself with healing moments. In the next chapter, we'll talk about ways to make sure that your visits are filled with healing moments.

CHAPTER 6

Healing Encounters: Tips on Creating Visits That Help You to Heal

Every interaction with a fellow human being has great potential for healing. If you're healthy, a visit with another person is a chance for both of you to become more whole, energized, and full of vitality. If you're ill, a visit is a golden opportunity for healing—for you and your visitor. Hospital visits give you a chance to maintain a connection with the outside world, including community, family, friends, and co-workers. They can be a time for reinforcing your spiritual practices, dealing with problems and fears, but also laughing, having fun, or singing.

If things went perfectly, visitors would always show up when you wanted company and never when you didn't, they'd always be the people you wanted to see, they'd act the way you wanted them to act, and they'd leave when you wanted them to leave. We can't promise you that level of perfection any more than we can promise you immortality—but we *can* guarantee that you and your visitors will have positive experiences as long as you all pay attention to your individual needs.

Too often, healing opportunities are lost because we're stuck with old misconceptions about what visits are all about, and you'll find that people will have all sorts of reasons for stopping by to see

you when you're ill. They may come out of love, concern, a desire
to be helpful, guilt, a sense of obligation, and many other motives.
In our estimation, the bottom line is always your healing, so there's
only one reason for people to visit right now—to help you to heal.
If everyone keeps their eyes on that goal, you'll have visits that will
also provide a lot of wonderful secondary benefits to everyone
involved. While your visitors are helping you, they can also contribute to their own well-being by nurturing feelings of love, and
by strengthening and deepening their relationship with you.

Don't forget that visits with pets are also important healing
opportunities. We know of a case where a dying person's dog was
brought to the intensive care unit (ICU) for a last good-bye. The
dog's licks, kisses, and contact brought the individual out of a
coma and changed that hospital's ICU visiting policy. Remember
that meaningful relationships are what keep us alive, including
those with animals. If you're fortunate enough to have beloved
pets, include them in your visiting plan—you'll find that they
always visit for the right reasons, and they never have to be taught
how to be *healing* visitors.

Managing Your Visits

Every visitor can help you in one way or another once you
learn how to manage your visits—the key is to make your needs
known. When your visitor is someone you don't want to talk to
intimately, ask him or her to read you stories, poems, or jokes;
massage your feet; help you write Vital Signs; or just sit and be
silent. If you have an overly talkative visitor, you can turn what
might have been an anxiety-producing imposition into a pleasant
respite by asking the person to do a silent meditation with you.
Remember that you're the only one who knows what feels right for
you, and as a respant, you need to dump the submissive-guy (or
gal) routine and let people know what your needs are.

Be aware that your visitors will bring along their own personal memories, hopes, and fears. When visitors enter the room and you've exchanged greetings, you may want to take a moment to remember that they arrived with psychological baggage. Try picturing them with actual luggage, such as a backpack full of emotions—what they're feeling right now and what emotional memories they have from past hospital experiences. Love your visitors for who they are and what they bring, but remember that their issues are *theirs,* not yours. Make sure that you see their baggage leaving with them. If necessary, you can explain that you don't need another visit if they can't leave some of their burdens at home, or if they're depleting your energy, hope, or spirit. If their behavior puzzles you, ask them to explain—understanding brings about forgiveness and a healthy dialogue.

If you've ever gone to see anyone at a hospital, then you have some experience to draw on in managing your visits. You'll be able to appreciate that your visitors may be nervous or scared, especially when they come to see you for the first time. The toughest part for them is usually crossing the threshold and walking into your room. They may not know what your health situation is, or whether it's okay to ask, and they'll probably be very worried about you. Seeing you may rekindle their own memories of hospitals and illnesses, and may evoke concerns about their own health and fears about their mortality. Their first words will give you the clue. If they ask, "How are you?" then they can deal with your answer. If they come in and say, "You look terrific," or "Isn't this a nice room?" then they may have difficulties, and may be hoping to avoid any emotional discussions.

Visitors are often uncomfortable simply letting interactions unfold naturally. They may be scared that they won't know the "right" thing to say or do. With the best of intentions, they often fall into whatever behavior they have in their mind for the role of "hospital visitor." If all they have to draw on is what they've seen other visitors do, then they probably won't know much about helping you to heal.

Maybe you'll be fortunate enough to have a friend who knows how to truly be "present" with you. More often, though, visitors believe that they're supposed to cheer you up, perhaps by denying everything that's going on, and assuring you that things will get better. Some will even expect you to engage in the denial and do the reassuring.

Beyond the other coaching tips we offer you and your loved ones, we can tell you one surefire way to have a healing visit with anyone: Be forgiving. Forgive every visitor, in advance, for everything he or she will do "wrong," or for behaving stupidly or awkwardly. Forgiveness is at the heart of loving, and loving is at the heart of healing. After all, life is a human comedy.

Tips on Having Visits That Help You To Heal

As you move through your hospitalization and convalescence, your visiting needs will change. At times you'll want visits from different people, and for different reasons. Some things will remain constant, though, and at every point in your convalescence, you'll need visitors who know how to be honest and authentic with you. You'll desire contact with people with whom you feel relaxed—those who are committed to helping you to heal.

In Chapter 11, we offer visitors some tips on how they can help you. Tell your friends about this chapter and ask them to read it—you'll be helping yourself and others at the same time. Your loved ones are likely to visit other people in the hospital in the future, and by becoming members of your empowered healing team now, they'll learn how to be healing visitors even for those who aren't respants and haven't formed a healing team.

You and your loved ones might try looking at visits as a dance. You're the one in most immediate need of healing, so you get to decide what kind of dance it will be and how long it will last. What will be the mood of your next dance? Will it be slow and intimate? Meditative and serene? You might prefer fast and funky, lively and fun, or mischievous and spontaneous.

Whatever mood you choose, you and your dance partner are healing partners, and the most important thing you can do is be yourselves. Don't let yourselves fall into the roles of "host," "guest," "caretaker/comforter," "wounded hero," "martyr," or "great pretender." No rehearsals are necessary when you stick to being your authentic self.

As a respant, you have just three responsibilities during a visit: (1) Be as comfortable as you can be, (2) make your needs known, and (3) let yourself be taken care of. For some of us, the third one is the most difficult. You may be reluctant to let others love and care for you, but what better time to give it a try? Everyone needs special attention when they're ill, so this is a wonderful chance to learn how to accept it. Stop being the strong one, and let someone rock you to sleep tonight.

You may even allow yourself to be pampered. What would make you feel indulged—a facial? A massage? Being read to? Having someone laugh at all your jokes? You may have found it hard to request these things under normal circumstances, but now that you're ill, it might be easier to ask for what you really want. Think about what hasn't been said that needs to be spoken, and do it.

Your visitor can help you in many ways. For example, he or she can:

- be a gatekeeper and keep intrusions and distractions away while you have downtime or white-room time, or while you do some of the healing work we'll talk about in the next chapter;

- create and post new Vital Signs, or help arrange your room (including bedding, plants, cards, and photos);

- see that you have an ample supply of Visitor Cards at the nurses' station;

- assist you with food, and with going to and from the bathroom;

- be your temporary personal-care attendant and do your hair or give you a facial; and

- shop for you and bring the items you need the next time he or she visits.

By letting people know what you need, asserting yourself, and referring your loved ones to the appropriate sections of this book, you can turn your visitors into healing partners. Be aware, though, that many people won't want to read about visiting or do the work of learning how to help you heal. But many *will* care enough—be prepared for some nice surprises as you discover which of your friends and acquaintances turn out to be your most helpful visitors.

Try some healing activities. If your visitor really wants to help you heal, he or she can join you in activities that support your inner life, meet your immediate needs and preferences, and give you a sense of control. Healing activities are good for getting love and warmth flowing—in both directions. You can pray or meditate together, you can read or share stories, and you can check out the menu of items we offer in "Healing Ways" (Part III).

Organize a visiting schedule. The timing of a visit can be almost as important as the quality of the visit, so talk with your family and friends about when you'd like visits. Encourage them to organize a schedule so that the pacing of their visits matches your needs. When you're thinking about how often you want company, make sure you pay attention to what your body is telling you. This is a time to respect your physical needs as well as your emotional, mental, and spiritual ones.

Don't spend your energy organizing the visits. Have someone on your team develop the schedule and communicate your needs to anyone who might stop by. As we mentioned in Chapter 3, someone can set up a Website or e-mail list to keep all of your friends up-to-date. The goal is to provide you with visits at times you choose, so you're not overwhelmed on Sunday afternoons and left alone on weekdays.

Your friends can also serve as a healing valet service, with the morning's visitors informing those coming in the afternoon what you'd like brought, or what errand you need someone to run. One visitor might take home some of your personal items to wash, and another might bring them back. Your loved ones will also benefit from this kind of organization because the care-taking burden will be shared. When you have well-organized visits, the people who care about you can feel secure knowing that you're being attended to and that everyone will have some quality time alone with you.

Only have visitors when you want company. It's easier to make visits work when you truly feel like having them. Keep in mind that you don't have to see anyone when you don't want to, and if you say no at times, then you'll feel a lot more joyful when you say yes.

Does it strike you as rude or offensive to decline a visit when someone has come to see you? Before you feel too guilty about saying no, ask yourself this: Would a thoughtful friend want to be with you when the time isn't right? If a person who truly cares about you arrives at an inappropriate time, he or she will want to honor your wishes and skip the visit rather than force you to act polite while you suffer in silence. It's not so hard to say no if you and your potential visitor remember that your mutual mission is your healing. Accept a hug, and off they go.

For those times when you don't want visits, you can use one of the signs you made at your prehospitalization Vital Signs party. If you didn't arrive with Vital Signs, then make one now. If you have a private room, then you can close your door and hang the sign outside the door. If you have a semiprivate room, pin the note to your cubicle curtain. Here's an example:

> *Thank you for coming—I need my rest right now.*
>
> *If you can, please call_____ at_____ to find out the best time to come back.*
>
> *I'd also appreciate it if you left a note for me on one of the cards I've provided at the nurses' station. Your visit is a source of healing and comfort for which I am very grateful!*

When we discussed preparations in Chapter 3, we talked about creating Visitor Cards that people can use when they arrive to find you resting or otherwise unready for visitors. If you made these cards, you can ask your nurse to keep them for you at the nurses' station. If you didn't, you can write some cards that say something like this:

Visitor Card

Patient's name_____
Thank you for caring. Sorry I wasn't able to see you.
Message:
Visitor's name [please print]_____

If you're not able to create these cards, then ask the nurses to tell your visitors when company isn't appropriate. They can suggest that your friends leave notes instead. If the nursing staff is too busy to intercept visitors, then make a sign and ask a nurse to tape it on your door or closed cubicle curtain.

If none of these methods feel right, you can always greet your friends and ask them to stay just a few minutes. Always let them know that you appreciate the effort they made, and in turn they'll appreciate your honesty in expressing your needs.

Yosaif: My late mother-in-law used to approach her days as if they were oranges, each moment being a sweet succulent drop of juice. Each day she aimed at getting every last drop of juice from that fruit.

By forgiving every visitor in advance for being less than perfect, and by using some of the coaching tips we've prescribed, you'll tap in to this reservoir of sweet healing nectar. Every visit is an opportunity for healing—our wish for you is that you enjoy every last drop.

As a respant, you can see whom you want, when you want, for as long as you want. Whatever the frequency and duration of visits, you can fill them with activities that help you to heal. In the next chapter, we'll look at some of the activities you can do in the long and important hours between visits, when you spend time with one of the nicest, wisest, most interesting people in your life—*yourself.*

ॐ

CHAPTER 7

Prescriptions for Self-Healing

Yosaif: Sol Alinsky, a well-respected community organizer, used to say that for every negative, there's a corresponding positive. When I was doing community organizing work in the 1960s, I'd sometimes walk the streets in search of that elusive positive. Sometimes it remained hidden, but other times I had the "Aha!" experience of discovering the good that balances the bad.

Bernie's mother taught a similar lesson when she always responded to problems by saying, "Something good will come of this." Alinsky and Bernie's mom are right: Corresponding positives come in many forms—even threats to your health contain blessings when they help complete your existence and lead you to discover truths about the nature of life.

One positive aspect you may have already discovered is the *time* you now have available. With your normal life on hold (or in the process of changing), and with confinement being imposed on you, you may find that another doorway is opening. This might be a passage back toward your inner life—a part of your being that you may have neglected while you dealt with the excessive busyness of your everyday life. But now you have the time to take care of yourself, and you may find that you can save your life by letting your untrue self die. Now you can stop being the person you became for everyone else's sake—when you're ill, you no longer have to be the "good kid" and conceal your feelings.

Whatever healing crisis you're undergoing right now, you can use your difficulties to grow spiritually and to renew yourself, or give yourself rebirth. Go through that open doorway, or that birth canal, and pay renewed attention to your inner life. This is as vital to your healing as anything else you can do, or that can be done for you now.

Please don't be put off by the mention of *spirituality* and *inner life*. When we use the terms *inner life, spiritual growth,* and *renewal,* we're not sermonizing. We recognize that your spiritual life may not involve religious practice, and we're not in the business of teaching or preaching about theology. We keep coming back to spiritual growth and renewal only because our years of experience have taught us time and again that patients facing life challenges do better when they can find meaning in their challenges and grow because of them. This kind of spiritual growth, whether it involves religion or not, helps heal lives; and a healed life may lead to physical recovery as well.

You may want to view the time you have alone as a time for "self-visiting." You've been given a rare opportunity to spend time with the most fascinating and important person you know. Think of the advantages of self-visiting: For one thing, you can be sure you'll only be talking about things that interest you, and if you're an attentive self-visitor, then you'll find that you have someone who really listens to what's going on with you.

So, what are you feeling right now? What's been left unspoken for too long? These are important questions, and you can put yourself on the road to healing by asking and answering them. As you go through this exercise, listen to yourself, and don't judge. It may help if you imagine what you'd say to a friend having the difficulties you're having. If you were his or her wisest, most intuitive confidant (and you might be), how would you handle what you're hearing? Could you simply listen and witness—nonjudgmentally? Would you have any suggestions about how to approach the issues your loved one is talking about?

Some topics you may want to address are:

- What are you yearning for? What are you hoping for or praying for?

- What do you fear? What are you worried about?

- What are you angry about?

- What are you excited about? What are you looking forward to?

- What do you need to confess? Whom do you need to forgive?

- Whom would you like to pray for?

- Whom can you love?

Also, don't forget to reflect on what you have to be grateful for right now. When you feel lousy, it might strike you as Pollyannaish to think about being grateful. So what? If you're willing to ask yourself the question, then you'll discover that even in the worst of moments there are some things in your life that clearly are wonderful. No matter how much else is going wrong, you can be thankful for these blessings.

Tips on Managing a Self-Visit

Just as you manage visits with other people, think about how you want your self-visit to go. Given how you're feeling right now, what kind of self-visit is right for you? Do you prefer a quiet, reflective, serene self-visit?

If so, here are a few coaching tips:

- Choose to have a "serenity break." Put an appropriate Vital Sign on your door or closed cubicle curtain.

- Close your eyes and follow your breathing for a minute or two.

- Do some inspirational reading, prayer, or meditation.

- Use a guided-imagery tape, or listen to some soothing music, spiritual songs, Tibetan healing-bowl sounds, or nature recordings on a CD or with a sound machine.

If you prefer a more active and lively self-visit, you may proceed differently:

- Choose one of the physical exercises in the "Healing Ways" section. Done in moderation, these exercises feel good and have the wonderful effect of increasing your vitality. They also quicken the pace of your healing and help you to feel, and be, more in control. (To ensure that the exercises and level of exertion are appropriate for you at this moment, check with your nurse or physical therapist.)

- If you feel like moving, try an "In-Bed Boogie." This can be as simple as putting on music you can't resist and starting to move. An In-Bed Boogie, despite its name, can be a lovely waltz or ballet.

Yosaif: My good friend Ellen Weaver suggested that my wife and I help my mother-in-law do "Bedside Ballet" moments after she suffered a stroke. We did, and it helped her on her road to recovery. The experience also sent me on the path toward writing this book.

Some form of In-Bed Boogie is almost always possible. If you're able to read this, then there's a good chance that you can move *something*—if not your fingers, hands, arms, legs, or pelvis, then your eyes, nose, mouth, tongue, or cheeks (those on your face *and* on your tush!).

Maybe you need to laugh with yourself. The time is almost always right for laughing, so play yourself a humor tape or read funny stories. Go for the ones that create the belly laughs that Norman Cousins called "internal jogging." That kind of laughter is good aerobic exercise. If you don't have stories or tapes available, watch a "movie of the mind"—in other words, remember scenes from movies or TV shows that had you rolling with laughter. Which ones work for you? Perhaps think of films or shows with Jerry Seinfeld, Chevy Chase, Gilda Radner, Eddie Murphy, Richard Pryor, Lily Tomlin, Robin Williams, Goldie Hawn, Mel Brooks, the Monty Python comedy troupe, Lucille Ball, or the Marx Brothers.

If you feel that your self-visit is a time for talking, then spend some time writing in a journal, which is self-talk in a written form. If you feel like drawing, try working from your dreams, thoughts, feelings, hopes, fears, and fantasies. Sketching this material is a powerful way to tap in to your own deep inner wisdom that will lead you onto a healing path.

We know that the hospital environment provides so many intrusions on your personal space that having a good self-visit can be difficult. While you're in the hospital, you may find that you're only able to spend short episodes of uninterrupted time alone. However brief these visits are, keep at it. Spending time with yourself is the most important thing you can do right now. Your healing—and your survival—may depend on whether you take the time to remove the lid from your treasure chest and let your unconscious wisdom express itself.

You can enhance your inner life and sense of personal control by setting aside a few minutes on rising and before going to sleep—the "bookends" of each day. Tell the nursing staff that your well-being depends on this, and ask for their support. Find out what time they need you to be awake in the morning, and keep an alarm clock (with gentle sounds or music) at your bedside so you can wake up by yourself 15 minutes early. If that's not feasible, try having someone on your healing team give you a wake-up call at the time you indicate. When you rise, take a few moments to do a brief meditation, visualization, or prayer. Don't forget to pray for the needs of your loved ones as well as for your own needs. You may choose to focus on your gratitude for being alive and being taken care of right now, or you may simply choose to lie there quietly, thankful that you woke up. You may also want to set your healing goal for the day. That way, by the time the hospital staff begins their morning routine and "hospital time" takes over, you've already risen on your own and experienced your wholeness (and holiness).

When you're ready to go to sleep, check with the nursing staff to see that they've completed everything they need to do for your care for the night. Then do a ritual similar to the one you did in the morning. Besides expressing gratitude, this is a particularly good time to express forgiveness toward yourself, your loved ones, the hospital staff, and your body. Let go of the toxins of anger and resentment, confess that you're only human, and release worry— at least for the night. If you can't fully let go of it, you can park it at your bedside and pick it back up in the morning if you need to. When you wake up the next day, you may find your problems are smaller and lighter, and you may decide to let the worry stay parked where it is.

The dictionary defines *vitality* as "the capacity for survival or for the continuation of a meaningful or purposeful existence; the power to live and grow." That's exactly what we want for you. We want you to have vitality in your life wherever you're convalescing. If you spend time engaged in healing activities while you're in the hospital, you won't fall into the role of submissive, suffering patient. Instead, you'll take control of your space and time, and create experiences that contribute to your "meaningful existence." You'll have the power to live and grow. Your Vital Signs, your visits with loved ones, and the activities you do on your own will keep you on a healing path, and soon you'll be ready to begin thinking about your next challenge: How to continue the healing process after you leave the hospital.

ॐ

CHAPTER 8

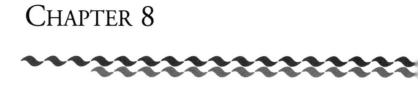

Getting Out: Continuing the Process of Healing

By now you're aware that you *can* have a healthy hospitaliza- tion—meaning that you can experience healing while you're in the hospital. When the time comes for you to be discharged, you can continue your healing by using the same respant approach that started you on a healing path in the first place.

People are sometimes frightened by the discharge process and the idea of being on their own again. However challenging their treatment has been, they're fearful of leaving the comfort and security they've enjoyed in the hospital. They think of going home (or to another facility) as akin to being set adrift, and they fear that they'll land in a scary, unpredictable world—feeling tired, weak, and very vulnerable. Anticipating such a miserable scenario, who'd ever want to leave the hospital?

These fears are not necessarily a problem for empowered patients, who are *en*charged rather than *dis*charged. Empowered patients stay in the hospital only as long as it serves their well- being, and then they leave to take the next important steps on their healing odyssey. Since they've known from the beginning that they have the right to leave the hospital, they've been making decisions about how long they need to stay all along.

Now, as you get ready to transition out of the hospital, you and your healing team can bring that same empowered awareness to charting the next part of your journey. Begin by asking yourself if this is the right time for you to leave. We don't mean, "Is this the right time, from your HMO's perspective, for you to vacate your bed?" We're asking, "Does your well-being require you to move on now? Or are you seeking to leave because you're not getting the care you require?"

A friend of ours, who is a doctor and a paraplegic, was unhappy with her treatment in the hospital. She asked to see her own doctor, but the nurse and resident physician wouldn't place the call—so she insisted on being discharged. Later, she wrote about her experience and explained why she'd asked for discharge despite being afraid to leave. "I felt powerless," she wrote. "They didn't even give me the respect of addressing me as an equal. I knew I'd be foolish to go home, but I just wanted to get out of there as fast as possible. I didn't want these people who didn't care about me acting as my physicians." Fortunately, the woman's primary doctor happened to be in the hospital seeing another patient that day, heard what was going on, and took over.

What our friend needed was attention, not a discharge. Had she been able to pick up the phone and make a call to her own doctor, she wouldn't have had to ask to be discharged when she wasn't ready.

Continuing the Healing Process

A healthy discharge takes planning—think of it as "transition planning." It's never too early to begin preparing: When you're making plans for a hospital stay for an elective procedure, you can also be making your post-hospitalization plans. Then, throughout your hospital stay, use your time to evaluate what you'll need in the next stage of your healing. Don't wait until the day of your discharge; take the time to incubate your thoughts and make the right choices. Discuss your ideas and options with your team and see what they think—but remember, *you're* the final judge.

On a practical level, what are some of the things you'll need to do to prepare for this next transition? The first task is deciding where you'll go when you leave the hospital. Ask yourself whether it makes sense at this point to go home and get some live-in or part-time help. Perhaps it's a better idea to move to an assisted-living facility, nursing home, rehabilitation hospital, or relative's home. Your decision can involve a number of steps—you may need extra care and attention for a while before you make the move to a more independent situation.

If you're going to another facility, then this is the time to use every resource possible to research your options and whittle down the choices. Think honestly about what's best for you and your care. Your financial situation, your health insurance, and your long-term care insurance may drive some of the choices you make, but talk to your team about all of the possibilities. You can also consult with experienced guides (such as discharge planners, social workers, case managers, family members, and informed and wise friends) who can help you chart your course. Tell them how you feel. If you're tired, let them know. If you're unable to visit the places on your list, ask team members to visit them for you and to evaluate the facilities.

Just as you used dreams and drawing to prepare for hospitalization, you can use them to prepare for the next part of your journey. Draw the choices you're considering. Your sketches speak the truth—they can help you understand how you feel, at an intuitive level, about your discharge. Use the information from your drawings and from the research you and your team members do, and then make the choices that feel best to you.

When you're ready to leave, don't abandon the healing progress you've made in the hospital. You don't have to stop being a respant just because you're leaving. Take your empowered identity with you wherever you go. Set up your photos and your bulletin boards, and keep expressing yourself. Let people know if you have disabilities, especially when they involve your sight, hearing, or ability to speak. And put Vital Signs on your door, just as you did in the hospital.

Continue exploring your healing alternatives. Learning about the range of traditional and complementary treatments and therapies was important while you were in the hospital, and it's even more important to integrate all these elements after you leave. Investigate any option that interests you, and anything you learn about from your healing team. You want to stay on a healing path.

Remember that your body responds to the healing messages you give it. Giving your body "live" and "heal" messages is just as important after you leave the hospital as it was when you arrived there. We've seen what happens when people are moved to new settings that they find depressing: When they're no longer exposed to beneficial therapies and they lose the sense of meaning in their lives, their recovery stops and they become vulnerable to further illness.

Many therapies are available to continue and enhance your healing process after you're discharged. Among them are acupuncture, guided imagery and hypnosis, massage, nutritional counseling, psychological counseling, qigong, reiki, reflexology, spiritual counseling, therapeutic touch, yoga, quiet walks, journaling, aromatherapy, music therapy, and more. The details of these techniques are available in books, on tapes, and via the Internet, but remember that just learning about them won't do you any good; information doesn't change you—change comes when you're inspired to take *action*.

If you're motivated and you want to be a survivor, then you'll explore your alternatives and try the ones that feel right to you. If one of the complementary therapies helps, continue it; if not, let it go. Don't worry too much about other people's beliefs about healing or their prescriptions for you. What matters is your experience with various treatments and healing modalities. Think of the techniques in the previous paragraph as items in a store—make your shopping list of therapies you want to try and add them to your healing plan.

Whatever you decide to try, remember the key lesson you learned while you were in the hospital: Healing is a process, not a product—a journey, not a single destination. When you're healed, your *body* isn't necessarily free of afflictions, but your *life* is.

You can help yourself heal by finding the rhythm that's right for you and establishing it in your life. This is a personal matter that's different for everyone: For example, some people need to live in the center of a vibrant city, while others need the serenity of nature. When you know your inner self, you'll know what's right for you.

Give yourself white-room time. This is especially important after discharge, because you may feel tired—sometimes for weeks—as your body uses your energy for healing. While you're convalescing, your body knows you need rest; it wants you to use your energy to heal your wounds and strengthen your immune system, so it sends you signs that your need to take a time-out. Remember that resting involves your psychology as well as your physiology, and you're not truly at rest if you don't have peace of mind. When you're worrying and visualizing the worst outcome, you're not allowing yourself any respite.

> **Bernie:** I had to learn an important lesson about rhythm. I used to think naps were a waste of time—why rest when I could be *doing* something? Then I hurt my back and realized that resting *is* doing something. Now I know that taking a break helps me to heal and restore myself, and this practice has become a part of my daily life.

To achieve peace of mind, you may need to settle your personal issues—ranging from emotional to financial. But when making decisions about your finances, remember that you're an important person who deserves care—don't deny yourself what you need because of the cost. Dying rich isn't a healthy goal to pursue. After all, you can't take it with you when you go. We can understand your wanting to leave something for your family, but your needs come first as long as you still have a will to live.

If you feel that you need to straighten out financial issues, then talk to your family or team members. If you don't have an accountant or attorney in the family, you may want to seek professional financial advice, or you (or a team member) may be able to find the information you need on the Internet. If you have an estate, you may need to retain an attorney who specializes in estate planning and trusts.

Family discussions about discharge plans and finances don't have to be difficult—they can actually be part of your healing. In responding to disease, you may find yourself discussing subjects you've never before confronted. This is part of the healing process, because unresolved problems can make you and others in the family sick.

Before You Leave

When the time comes to leave a facility where you've been cared for, thank everyone who has touched your life in a meaningful way. This may include the people who brought your meals and emptied your wastebasket, as well as those who performed major surgery. Remember that no one is free of difficulties, and everyone healing you has his or her own wounds. Show your appreciation to your wounded healers. Give people who help you to heal a button that says, "You Make a Difference."

Thank-yous don't have to be one-time messages. On the anniversary of your discharge, you can go back to visit the hospital or send a card saying "Thank you again." Hospital workers care for one sick person after another, many of whom they can't cure. In the process, they tend to forget all the people they've helped. When you express your gratitude and remind them of how they aided you, you're helping them to heal as well.

Self-Defense Against Post-Discharge Medical Errors

Unfortunately, medical errors don't stop happening when you leave the hospital. There should be a sign over the exit warning, "Caution: Only you can prevent yourself from becoming a post-discharge medical error!" Researchers at the Harvard Medical School and the University of Ottawa found that 76 of the 400 post-discharge patients they interviewed had "adverse events" after discharge. The researchers discovered that the most common adverse events were due to medication errors, and that with better communication between doctors and patients, and between doctors themselves, two-thirds of these errors could have been prevented.

Dr. David Bates, one of the researchers from Harvard, told us, "I think it's very important for patients and families to know what the medications they're taking are, to know something about the side effects of the medications, and—most important—to let their provider know if they begin to experience a bothersome new symptom. In our research, we've found that patients often wait too long to contact their provider."

Don't wait for your physicians to learn better communication skills in their continuing education courses. Act now in self-defense to improve your odds of avoiding such "adverse events."

- Ask your hospital doctor(s) to e-mail your diagnosis, case history, and treatment to your referring physician (and to send you or a family member a copy, too).

- Call your doctor if you have any questions about taking the prescribed medications (especially if you're having reactions), or about anything you need to know about your own care. If your doctor doesn't respond to your call, just remember that it's your health and your life; don't be afraid of being seen as a "problem." Having problems doesn't make *you* the problem.

Planning for the Final Transition

We have one more important issue to deal with in contemplating discharge plans and transitions. We've heard from many people who believe that the way to escape from what's killing them is to end their lives. If you're thinking this way, know that it's a lot healthier and more sensible to eliminate what's destroying your life, release what has been burdening you, and free yourself to create a *new* life for yourself. On the other hand, we also know that for each of us, there will come a time when it's no longer a joy to reside in our body.

> **Bernie:** One day, my father told my mother, "Rose, I need to get out of here." She thought he was talking about his hospital bed, but he was actually referring to how he felt about living in his disabled body.
>
> A similar sentiment was expressed to me by the father of a dying child, "Our job as parents, doctors, and teachers isn't to defeat death, but to defeat the pain of living." It's only when we accept our mortality that the true process of healing can begin. When we accept the fact that we're going to die, then we discharge ourselves from all the baggage we drag through life, which retards our healing.
>
> While you're accepting your mortality and letting go of your burdens and your baggage, you can even plan your own funeral. Some of the most vibrant, full-of-life people I know have made their own final arrangements, picking out the music, caterer, and clergy for the event. They love doing that planning. Sometimes, when you get all the preparations done and you speak about what was unspoken, you feel so good that you become a hospice dropout!
>
> Thinking about how much death has taught me and my patients, I wrote this poem, called "The Great Teacher."

Death, what a great teacher you are
Yet few of us elect to learn from you about life
That is the essence of death's teaching
Life
Death is not an elective
One day we all will take the class
The wise students audit the class in early years
And find enlightenment
They are prepared when graduation day comes

I know a dying man who wrote in his journal that as he approached the inevitable end of his life, time became more valuable—much more valuable than money. When you think about your death, you know that the cliché "Time is money" is simply wrong. Time isn't money; time is *everything*.

If you think about the end of your life, you'll realize that seeing something for the last time is just as good as seeing it for the first time. You'll see the wisdom in giving even more love to those who love you, and devoting yourself less to those who don't care about you. When you live with an awareness of your death, you're discharged from the absurdity we call life. You're free to begin living.

If you think about your mortality and accept it while you're convalescing, you'll be ready for anything. Then, if you're fortunate enough to leave the hospital alive, you'll find that you're ready to live more fully than ever.

ॐ

CHAPTER 9

Healing at Home:
Staying Empowered

Your healing journey doesn't have to end when you're well enough to return home. In fact, you can begin the process of healing at home now by taking a few minutes to answer some questions, such as:

- What does healing at home mean to you?

- Can you continue to recover by focusing attention solely on your physical and mental needs, or will your healing involve your relationships, too?

- Do you live alone, or with others? If you live with others, how do the relationships in your home affect you?

- When you're home and surrounded by caregivers, to whom do you reach out?

- What do you do when you have a problem and you can't handle it alone?

- Do you use your illness to manipulate or control your relationships?

Did you imagine being by yourself when you were answering the questions? In our view, you may be home alone, but you never have to be lonely because there's always a healing energy and awareness available to you. Learning about the healing energy is part of our PMS (**p**ractical, **m**ystical, and **s**piritual) plan for making transitions.

There is a consciousness and an awareness that exists always and everywhere—the name you give it is unimportant. Everyone is capable of experiencing this awareness, and each person's understanding of it will be unique. We're not talking about religion here; we're simply pointing you toward a resource that's available to you when you feel alone. If you take time to meditate about your life and your difficulties, and open yourself to the awareness, you'll feel this universal field of consciousness.

Bernie: I recently took a class in philosophy and religion. For the final exam, the professor gave each of us a live chicken and told us to kill it where no one would be aware of the act. At the next class, the students were all laughing because I brought my chicken back, still alive. I hadn't been the brightest student in the class that semester, so my classmates figured I'd misunderstood the assignment or hadn't been able to bring myself to do the deed.

The professor quieted the class and began calling on students to tell how they'd killed their chickens. One by one, the students talked about the elaborate plans they'd made and the secluded areas they'd found. At last, no one was left but me. The professor called my name and I took my chicken up and handed it to him, explaining, "I looked everywhere, but there was no place I could kill this chicken, because there's no place where there isn't any awareness of my actions."

The professor nodded, smiled, and gave me an A.

Psychologist Carl Jung talked about relying on your own resources when you encounter problems you can't solve. He said that you must have the courage to pay attention to a helpful idea or intuitive hunch, and to notice thoughts you'd previously ignored. Jung's advice certainly applies to the problem of finding a healing path. If you have the courage to look within and to trust your deeper nature, powers will emerge and intervene in your life.

"Helplessness and weakness are the eternal experience and the eternal problem of mankind," Jung acknowledged, but also pointed out that there must be solutions to our problems or humans wouldn't have survived. The search for answers takes us into the unconscious, and prayer is one way of connecting with our buried or unconscious wisdom.

If you don't know how to pray, try praying for the *ability* to pray, or reciting the alphabet and letting a higher source put the right words together. If praying makes you uncomfortable, you can take a similar journey by meditating, listening, and opening yourself to the resources, strength, and answers already present in your unconscious. When you begin to listen, you'll agree that you're never alone—no matter where you are.

Arranging Your Home for Healing

Now for the practical part of our PMS plan for transition. When you return home, you'll have the wonderful experience of seeing things with fresh eyes. This is a great opportunity for conducting what we call a "How does this help me heal?" survey. This survey is simple and straightforward. Most things will jump right out at you, and you'll wonder why you hadn't seen them before. Actually, you probably have seen them, but your mind deposited them in the "Who's got the time to deal with that?" file.

Now *you* have the time—and since you're in a healing frame of mind, you might even feel entitled to have a more supportive space in which to live. Other than feng shui experts and interior designers, most of us don't organize our living space with our well-being in mind. Most people live in environments that are, to a large extent, creations of happenstance reinforced by habit. Where you set things down when you first come into the house is where they're likely to remain. For example, what's the path a newspaper follows after it enters your home? How, in hospital parlance, is it "discharged"?

> **Yosaif:** In my house, newspapers stack up (often unread) and become small nagging piles of unfinished business. They're not discharged until they become such a nuisance that either my wife or I can't stand them anymore.
>
> If we were away for a while and returned home in a healing frame of mind, we might realize that it isn't good for us to be surrounded by piles of unread papers. Once we saw that, it would be easy enough to figure out a simple daily plan to remove this minor hindrance from our lives and replace it with clear space.

You'll have many practical matters to consider when you return home. If you're facing an extended convalescence in which you'll face physical challenges, you may need a discharge planner or a physical therapist to help you identify and solve problems: Will stairs be an issue? Are the bathrooms accessible? Do you have to climb into the bathtub to bathe? How easy is it to turn lights on if you get up at night? Who will prepare your meals? Do you need a call pendant (a small device worn around the neck that can alert authorities in case of an emergency)? Take the time to think through a typical day and anticipate what problems you might encounter.

If necessary, you can have your home redone by installing ramps or railings, or by adding motion-sensor lights. If that's too costly or time-consuming, consider going to a transition home first. This could be a health-care facility or the home of a friend or relative.

Some problems are difficult to anticipate, so you'll have to be alert as you go along.

Bernie: When my father-in-law became quadriplegic due to a fall, he spent time in a wheelchair and was unable to sit up straight. The family tried to work out a way of supporting him, but he'd slump forward and end up looking at people's feet. He found it depressing not to be able to see people's faces, but he didn't tell anyone and we weren't aware of the problem until a therapist visited one day and told us about wheelchairs with adjustable backs that enable the occupant to look up. This seemingly small change made an enormous difference in my father-in-law's life.

You can find many products designed to help seniors or disabled people deal with the challenges they face every day. When you realize that some facet of daily life is difficult, ask for help in finding the products or solutions that address the particular problem.

Be creative in thinking about what you'll need in order to heal at home.

Yosaif: A few years ago, my wife, Tsurah, had surgery and was facing an extended convalescence. We talked about her healing and the fact that our bedroom is right next door to my office, and we quickly realized that she wouldn't be able to convalesce with phones ringing, lights on at all hours, office equipment humming, and my prancing back and forth. Tsurah needed a serene, healing cocoon.

I'd chosen the space next to the bedroom for an office because it has a commanding view of the Ashokan Reservoir and the Shawangunk and Catskill Mountains. The view from the office inspired me and made me feel optimistic, which was helpful to my work. However, life goes on, and our needs were shifting. Now the most important thing in our lives was Tsurah's full and complete healing, and that could be disrupted by the activity in the office. She needed a bedside healing sanctuary where she could have control over her time and space. So I moved my office to the other side of the house, and interestingly enough, I wound up enjoying my new space, which was womblike and inspiring in its own way. The new office allowed me to concentrate more on my work, and also provided me with a place to play music as loud as I liked without disturbing Tsurah.

We made other changes, too—including installing a new telephone line. That way, at the beginning of her home convalescence, Tsurah could have her regular calls answered by our phone service, but our grown children and I were able to reach her on a private, unlisted line in our bedroom.

If you're returning home for a short convalescence, you'll want to focus most of your efforts on the space where you'll be spending the majority of your time. You may choose to get rid of clutter and make other changes that will be lasting to make you more comfortable. If you don't have a place in your home where you can be peaceful and serene, this is the time to create one—even if it's a small nook in your bedroom. A water fountain and a candle can create an instant sanctuary, as can a poster with a scene from nature and relaxing music. You may want to go further and fill the space with pictures, symbols, and items that evoke pleasant memories. This will be the place you can go when you need rest or when you need to restore yourself, so tell everyone that your sanctuary is a sacred spot and isn't to be violated.

As you're paying attention to the sights and sounds throughout your home, take a moment to think about the scents, too. Studies have shown that some aromas give people a sense of well-being. Most doctors aren't aware that our sense of smell can have such a powerful effect on us, but real estate agents know it and use fragrances to sell houses. So fill your space with comforting scents, such as vanilla or apple pie.

In addition to spending time in your healing sanctuary each day, you can resume creative pastimes, such as writing poems and letters or doing projects around the house. Activities that make you lose track of time are especially good for helping you to heal, so do as much as feels right to you. But remember that any activity that you *don't* want to do won't help you heal. Work isn't a healing activity—unless you love your work so much that it makes you lose track of time, because in that case (by our definition) it's not work.

Make a point of going outside every day, weather permitting. Just as pictures of natural scenes helped you to heal while you were in the hospital, observing nature outside your home will help you recover faster and experience less pain. If you live in an apartment building facing a brick wall, it's even more important that you try to get out for a power walk or ride. Don't be embarrassed to go out in a wheelchair, use a cane, or wear a bandage—what your neighbors think isn't important; your recovery is your greatest concern, and time outside is invigorating. Plus, you may find that if you don't hide your wounds, your neighbors will reveal theirs to you, and your outdoor time will become group therapy.

Arranging Your Time for Healing

While you're preparing to heal in your home, you'll want to consider time as well as space. Think about the kind of caring attention you'll require, and talk about your concerns with your team. Discuss the schedule each person in your home will follow, and find out who can help you with each need. For example, who will keep track of your medications? Who will make your meals and change your dressings? Will someone be home at all times? Are you well enough to be alone for part of the day? If you're not, look for help from an agency, or consider asking a neighbor. You must be willing to ask for assistance when you need it, and you don't know who can help unless you ask. When you do ask someone for help, you're doing them a favor, because you're giving them an opportunity to feel good about being of service to others.

Pets can be healing companions, but they can also pose problems while you're convalescing. Who will walk the dog, clean the cat's litter box, and take the animals to and from the vet? This may not have been a problem before, but now you may need someone to provide care for them as well.

Make it easier for your teammates to help you by writing a list of tasks that need to be done: housecleaning, shopping, pet care, and so forth. Ask them to meet and discuss their schedules and let them decide how they can help best. You don't have to work this all out by yourself. If the sight of blood makes one of your visitors ill, he won't volunteer to change your dressing or hold your hand when the technician comes to draw blood—but he may be the perfect person to tend your houseplants.

You don't have to become a recluse because you're confined—but you don't have to be a great host, either. You decide who you are and what you need for yourself in the way of contact with other people. If you can, use your healing tag team to let people know when you want or need visits. You probably don't want everyone showing up the first weekend you're home, so you'll need to manage your visits just as you did in the hospital. It might sound funny, but if people you know are dropping by without calling first, you can resurrect your Vital Signs to control the traffic and make these visits satisfying and rewarding. You can post signs on your door or place them strategically around the house—such as on the refrigerator or bathroom door.

Your telephone can also either be a healing gift or a destructive drain on your energy. Just remember that *you* make the decisions—the telephone doesn't. When you want time to rest, take the phone off the hook or turn the ringer off. Likewise, if you have an e-mail account, you don't need to check it every hour. We guarantee you that the world won't end if you don't read your e-mail, open your snail mail, or answer your telephone for one day. If you don't believe us, then try it and see what happens. If this makes you uncomfortable, put automatic messages on your answering machine and computer to let people know when you'll be responding.

You can even transform everyday sights or sounds—stop signs, red lights, or the ringing of telephones—into calls to mindfulness. Use them as reminders that it's time to pause a moment to restore your wholeness.

Bernie: As I mentioned in Chapter 3, the telephone can be a real drain on your energy if you rush to answer it every time it rings. When someone calls me, I don't answer the phone for at least three rings. During those rings, I breathe peace for myself and for the person on the other end of the line. Try this, and then listen to the calm in your voice when you answer and the caller is an aluminum-siding salesman. You won't even mind, because he's just given you a peaceful healing moment.

If you plan on using the telephone in this way, be sure to inform your relatives so that they don't worry when you don't answer immediately. I called my 94-year-old mother the other day, and she didn't pick up the phone right away. When she finally did, I said, "Mom, are you okay? Why didn't you answer the phone?"

"I'm following your suggestion," she said.

"Mom, that advice is for everyone else," I explained. "*You* need to answer the phone on the first ring so that I don't worry!"

Now she picks up right away for me and meditates on her own time.

Staying Empowered

Beyond all the physical changes you make when you return home, don't forget to look for new opportunities to care for your soul and spirit. You didn't live a role in the hospital—so don't do it at home, either. Be your authentic self and make sure that your home environment supports you in every way possible.

Your empowerment doesn't have to end when you return home. Here, just as in the hospital, your health may depend on your:

- awareness of your own strengths and limitations;

- willingness to set boundaries and take time for self-nourishment; and

- sensitivity to your own personal signs of stress.

If you want to continue to heal, then maintain your respant behavior by:

- being a responsible participant in your own healing;

- developing strategies for handling grief and loss;

- finding and maintaining balance in your life; and

- building a good support system.

We have one final and important point for you to consider, respantly: *Is your home still your home?* Is it, in Robert Frost's words, " . . . the place where, when you have to go there, they have to take you in"? For most of us, home is a place filled with a lifetime of memories and emotional experiences. Do your memories evoke pleasant and happy thoughts, or are they painful? Were your emotional experiences damaging? If your home environment contributed to your illness, and returning there is going to bring up destructive, negative, draining thoughts, then go somewhere else. Your home should be a sanctuary, not a place where you relive physical or psychological abuse—past or present.

Unfortunately, home is a prison for some people. If that's your situation, then use your illness to free yourself and to guide you to a healing environment where people care about you. You *can* find such a place. Remember, you're never alone or unloved.

❧

So far we've been talking about how *you* can be a respant—a responsible participant in your own care—and we've emphasized the importance of teamwork in healing. In Part II, we'll offer tips and coaching on how family, friends, and other caregivers can be effective members of your healing team. Read this next section yourself, and then show it to other members of your team who want to know how they can help you to heal.

෴

PART II

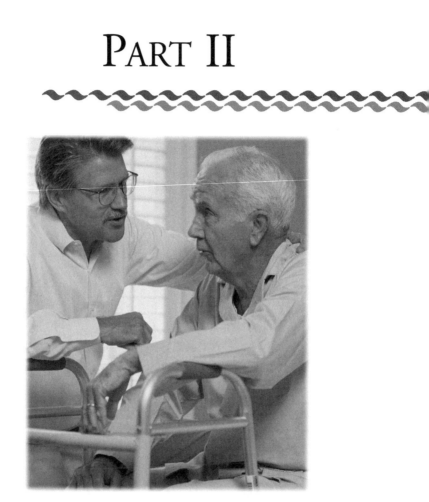

Healing Strategies for Family, Friends, and Caregivers

CHAPTER 10

Being an Empowering Advocate

The time may come in each of our lives when we're no longer in any condition to act on our own behalf. Even if we're respants, we're still mortal—and sometimes we need to be taken care of. When we reach this point, "Help me to heal" becomes a plea for someone to take the lead in assisting us, and the person who steps up to the plate is an advocate. Although we may all have different needs, what we'll ask of our advocate boils down to: "Please do everything you can to promote my healing."

Anyone can be an advocate. In fact, *you* may need to provide care for a loved one, friend, or family member someday—perhaps you're already doing so. If you're a health-care worker, from time to time you may find yourself representing patients who are in your care. The coaching tips in this chapter are designed to help you become an effective advocate—no matter how you're connected to the person you're trying to help.

Your role as an advocate depends on the needs of the patient. Some patients never choose to become empowered themselves, and they want someone to make decisions that are appropriate for them when they can't do so on their own. Those who are inspired by our healing philosophy may want to be in full control of their own healing, but they may need you to step in and take charge of their care temporarily. As their strength returns, they can assume more and more of their own advocacy, although they'll probably still welcome your support.

In our view, the best advocate is one who's *empowered* and *empowering*. This type of advocate will:

- act as the patient would want to act if able to represent him/herself;

- be empathetic—that is, try to understand how the patient perceives what's going on, and react accordingly;

- show respect for the patient's dignity, judgment, privacy, and autonomy;

- continually assess the patient's ability and willingness to assume partial or full advocacy on his or her own behalf;

- act to mobilize all caregivers—professionals, friends, and family—as a team that focuses on the patient's healing and comfort; and

- continually guard the patient's interests, expectations, preferences, and needs—and make sure that all caregivers are focused on the same goals.

If you're advocating for an "I don't care" patient, then you get to be the one who *does* care. You'll decide how much you need to micromanage things, or whether it's best to take a more relaxed approach. If you're advocating for a patient who knows exactly what she wants and how she wants it, then you'll support her in whatever way is necessary, and you'll be sure to express her desires. As an empowering advocate, you'll carry out her will, help her to be more in control of the situation, and never make her feel like a failure.

An empowering advocate can be helpful in any setting and at any time—from a doctor's office to an emergency room, from same-day surgery to a nursing-home stay. Wherever the care is being provided, your task is the same: to express the patient's will and get her the healing help she needs, while remembering that it's her disease and you need to allow her responsibility for it.

Bernie: Michael and Barbara Tucchio attend a weekly support group that I facilitate. The group offers assistance to facing illness or health challenges. It often happens that when introductions are going on, the advocates avoid sharing their feelings—they say that they're just "The Chauffeur." Mike wrote this, and I feel that it shares what all advocates need to understand: Patients and advocates are on a journey *together,* sharing the experience of healing.

In our 37th year of marriage, we shared a life-
    changing event
But an impossible 50-50 sharing, as all our pre-
    vious trials have been
How can we split this burden, based on our
    experiences of the past?
No, this will be a new paradigm, unlike any we
    have known

On that day in August, she came home from the
    doctor's exam,
The groin lymph nodes were enlarged, very visi-
    ble in the soft skin
Only two possibilities as I drove my investigation
    on the Internet,
The first is benign infection, the second an
    unknown cancer

This is not the time for vengeance, but for clear
    pursuit to gather information
Barbara and I will bring all our energies to bear
    on the intruder
We will wrestle with the information, see the
    facts, consult cancer sources,
List the statistics and find the protocols to com-
    bat the ugly enemy

The numbers are grim, the protocols many, a
    completely confusing array
What can we do to make the best of a very frus-
    trating, scrambled position?
We can read and find out what others did to
    make them survivors
Yes, there is something she can do—whatever it
    takes to be a survivor

But I am separated from my wife's reality, the
    cancer is in her body, not mine
Like the glass that separates the limousine driver
    from the passenger
The two occupants travel together
But I am only the chauffeur

Her new physicians are impressive—they actually
    talk to us and give important information
We feel a newfound confidence and drive ahead
    with vigor
Our daughters, Teresa and Danna, help discuss
    the situations and options
They provide solid footing, they are with us, as
    we meet with the docs and staff

So the chemotherapy has started to reduce the
    tumors to an operable size
And we commute to Providence, Rhode Island
    once a week, and it's obvious
We must make an essential decision, a key to our
    plan, a way of life
Barbara will do whatever she must to be the sur-
    vivor, and I will do the rest

My part-time job, running my little consulting
    company winds down
Household chores fill any spare moments that
    I may have
Somehow this doesn't seem like work but only
    my contribution
Someone once said to me, "It's what you do
    when you said, 'I do'"

We are a team. Two people with a singular goal;
    I will keep her world positive
Maintain the rudder in position or change our
    course when necessary
We live in the moment and catch the cool
    breezes or the warm sun
Whatever direction leads us to our goal

Our faith must provide the ingredient to tip the
    balance in her favor
We attend the healing mass at our church—the
    priest lays hands on her
She adds her hands on his and presses them to
    her head
A bond was formed at a time I knew, and noth-
    ing could be better

My cooking must be good, for by spring she put
on some weight,
Her muscles very gradually appeared, waiting to
be used
Even her breasts were fuller now, evident in her
building breath
Of lungs that were abused by malignant liquid
that was reaching within her chest

Her body is getting stronger, and by spring she is
in the garden
Planting the flowers that she cherishes so much
A symbol of life so precious that needs her loving
care, and more important
A life over which she can exercise control

Summer of 2001, and she is swimming—she
loves water sports
And then, late in July, on a chemo day, she is
waterskiing again
Oh, what a wonderful feeling for Barbara,
Danna, Teresa, and me
Oh, what a lust for life that has swelled up in her

It is now over two years and the fight continues
How proud I am of her—she has become a
symbol to many cancer survivors
She extends her experiences to them openly and
completely
She is educating whomever she can touch

I am the chauffeur; Lord, thank You for Your
guidance
Help me to cast positive energy through the
glass barrier

Father, focus Your love and compassion
  on Barbara
It is in Your hands that we may resume our
  journey side by side

Preparing for Advocacy

Before you decide to take on the role of advocate, stop and ask yourself some questions: Do you have a genuine calling to do this work, or are you becoming an advocate for unhealthy reasons such as guilt or ego? Are you stepping forward out of devotion and a deep connection with the person who needs an advocate? Answer honestly, and you'll know whether or not to become an advocate.

If you choose to take on this responsibility, then remember that you'll be better able to help others if you're living a healed life yourself. When you're truly prepared, you can be a source of calm in the storm; when you're not, your attempts to help may end up causing additional problems and disrupting the patient's recovery.

If somebody you care about needs an advocate and you don't feel prepared, then let someone else do the job—that is, if someone else is available. If not—if you and the patient are "stuck with" each other—then just do your best to be empathetic and empowering. It may help to remember that the past is over, and your challenge now is to live in the moment and provide whatever is needed. You may find that a by-product of becoming a loving advocate is a healing of past wounds.

If, however, you do the best you can and your relationship is still having a negative effect on your partner's health, then stop trying to advocate for him or her. You're not being effective if you're draining the patient's energy.

If you said yes to this role, then you can begin by tackling the items on the following list. It was originally written for professional-care managers, but it's appropriate for anyone who takes on advocacy out of love:

- Make an assessment of the patient's situation and needs.

- Create a care plan.

- Find and secure all the necessary services—from legal advice to convalescent care to home maintenance.

- Prepare to support and counsel the patient—as well as members of the family and healing team.

- Listen to what the patient is saying.

This last item—listening—might be the most important of all. As you go about your advocating, keep in mind the story a doctor wrote about the last patient he saw in his office one wintry Friday evening. The patient had a chronic illness and many complaints, but her doctor didn't have the patience to sit and listen to her. So he wrote her a prescription, quickly left the examining room, and put on his coat to go home.

When he got into his car, it wouldn't start. He went to a garage across the street, not really expecting much help since it was late on a snowy Friday. To the doctor's surprise, however, the mechanic was sympathetic and agreed to work on the car that weekend. In the meantime, the mechanic offered the use of a four-wheel-drive vehicle. He even went out into the snow to warm up the loaner for the doctor.

As he drove home in the borrowed car, the doctor realized that the mechanic had given him much better care than he had given his patient. He thought about the woman who'd needed to talk with someone about her losses and her problems, and he promised himself that from then on he'd practice four-wheel-drive medicine.

It's easy to understand why patients let their doctors and other health-care workers get away with acting like the doctor in this story. If you were a patient, would you want to raise hell with the hospital staff over an unmet need, knowing that you might have an emergency at 2 A.M.? What if the people on duty are the same people you bellowed at earlier? Will they come and care for you? Will they respond or just let you suffer? If you were in a hospital or nursing home and were dependent on others for care, raising troublesome issues would be scary, and you might be tempted to remain submissive—even if that meant receiving less-than-adequate care.

As an advocate, one of the most valuable things you can do is to speak up when the patient is afraid to, so that you're seen as the troublemaker and the patient isn't. But before you can speak up, you must take the time to listen. Good advocates don't try to be productive and detached like the doctor was when he dismissed his complaining patient—good advocates are empathetic.

> **Bernie:** In my father-in-law's record at his nursing home, there was an entry that said, "Son-in-law creating a problem." Why was I creating a problem? Because they were sedating a quadriplegic man whose forehead itched! I wanted them to scratch his forehead instead of using drugs to turn him into a vegetable. My father-in-law was afraid that if *he* complained about the itch, then the staff might not help when he needed them—and he was totally dependent on them for his every need. So I became his advocate and spoke for him, and I was a problem—but he wasn't.

What an Advocate Needs to Know

A coaching newsletter we received began with this observation: "The best athletes are coach-oriented, but not coach-dependent." In our years of experience, we've observed that the best patients are doctor- or advocate-oriented, but not doctor- or advocate-dependent.

The advocate/patient partnership is a two-sided relationship that depends largely on mutual trust. As an advocate, you're responsible for making judgments with honesty and certainty. But in order to do so, you have to believe in what you're doing. You have to have faith in the patient's dedication and commitment to healing decisions, be aware of any unique needs, and keep them in mind when trying to make big decisions. Your mind needs to work in concert with the patient's—you must be able to identify changes in the patient's physical and mental health and react to those changes by adjusting the healing plan. You may also need to modify the type of advocacy you practice as the patient's needs evolve.

To do your job well, you must educate yourself about all available sources of healing, and figure out how to weave them into a master plan that helps the patient progress with minimal risk. You need to understand the patient's medical needs, but remember that they're his needs and not yours. You and others on the healing team may prescribe treatments or therapies, but it's up to the patient to decide which prescriptions to fill.

> **Bernie:** When my father was very ill, I supported a treatment that I felt would help him. After it was done, he asked, "If you knew it was going to hurt that much, would you still have advised me to go through it?" It pained me to see him suffer, but nonetheless, I could honestly say that I would have chosen the treatment if I were in his place, and I genuinely believed it was right for him, too. If I thought that the treatment had been a mistake, I would have said so, because honesty is vital in the advocate/patient relationship . . . as it is in all relationships.
>
> Remember that advocacy is not a contest about who's right. As an advocate, you're still human and you're going to make mistakes, so be prepared to say, "I'm sorry, I was wrong."

It's important to know your patients' bill of rights, and make sure that all the caregivers and team members know it, too. If malpractice occurs or financial problems arise, be prepared to step forward and make decisions. Sometimes a patient might need to consider a lawsuit, but be aware that legal action won't heal emotional wounds, even when there's a successful outcome. Nonetheless, the patient's interests should be protected.

Often the fact that a patient has a strong advocate will be enough to resolve problems with a doctor, insurance company, or health plan. When it comes to health care and legal rights, the squeaky wheel does get the grease. For any minor problems that may arise, make sure that the respant you're advocating for has a Siegel kit available to help him call attention to his needs when you're not there.

When it appears that a hospital stay may be prolonged, you may want to form an advocacy team so that you don't become drained by the solo effort. Remember, advocacy that's not done out of love can make you feel resentful, and can end up doing more harm than good—you'll either burn up or burn out. These are different problems that respond to different cures, so if you're burning up, you may be restored by getting some rest; while if you're burning out, you won't feel better until you change your life—which may require either stepping down as advocate or bringing in other teammates to help you.

Your role as advocate continues through discharge and beyond. We talked in the last chapter about having a post-discharge healing plan, and you need to be involved in that planning. You should be with the patient at the time he or she checks out of the hospital to listen to the advice and information given by the nurses and doctors. If outpatient care is recommended, you can help organize transportation and make sure that someone will be available during the day to help with any follow-up care.

When you take on advocacy, you need to be willing to face one very emotional moment—especially if you're advocating for an older patient or someone who's very ill. Prepare yourself for the possibility that the person you represent may at some point say, "I'm tired and don't want to go on with treatment."

Athletes retire, and we will, too, eventually. For all of us, there may come a time when our bodies function so poorly that residing in them isn't truly living anymore. If the person you advocate for is at that point, you'll need to speak up for him. Help the family and medical staff understand that his death doesn't make them failures, and gently urge them not to prolong his dying to assuage the problems they may have with his death. Encourage people to say what needs to be said and to heal old wounds so that the patient can die in peace, surrounded by loved ones who can accept what's happening. We're writing to *in*spire you, but there may come a time when it's appropriate to *ex*pire.

When you suffer the loss of a loved one whom you've been an advocate for, be sure to use your pain to help others heal from their grief. We all become healers when we share our wounds and compassion in the service of love. Acknowledging your feelings and helping others acknowledge theirs is healthier than staying isolated or remaining numb or medicated. Blessings come in many forms—and it sometimes helps to remember that we wouldn't appreciate the light if we didn't experience periods of darkness.

If a patient dies in the hospital, then you and other team members may want to thank the staff for being there during trying times. However brief their contact with your loved one was, it was authentic. Your loss is a loss for them, too. Health-care practitioners rarely discuss their pain, but you can help them learn to acknowledge grief. Invite them to the funeral.

Of course you didn't *want* to lose your loved one, but sometimes the experiences that you don't want are the very ones that force you to search for meaning. Remember: Life is a series of beginnings.

Advocating for Younger and Older Patients

When you're advocating for a child, make sure that she knows the people who will be taking care of her. If possible, have her meet the medical personnel ahead of time so that she won't be frightened when it's time for treatment. Be sure to bring along toys, stuffed animals, games, and other items the child is comfortable with to distract her and alleviate her symptoms and fears, and don't be afraid to be silly. Finally, remember that empowerment is as important for kids as it is for adults—you can help a child feel empowered by giving her choices such as, "Would you like to climb up onto the examining table, or should we lift you?"

When a child trusts you, your words can have hypnotic power. We know a little boy who didn't lose any hair while on chemotherapy, because his parents changed the label on his vitamin bottle and began giving him "Hair-Growing Pills." Don't be afraid to deceive a child—or an adult—into health. We're not talking about lying, but about choosing to provide hope in the face of uncertainty. Remember, even a blind squirrel finds an acorn now and then.

If you're advocating for an older patient, then one of the best things you can do is to let her know that she's needed. Tell her about your problems and family issues, and ask for her advice based on her wisdom and years of experience.

> **Bernie:** My mother worries about herself when her advocate is unavailable—until she hears about the problems the advocate's family is having. Then she refocuses on helping her advocate heal, and her own worries diminish.
>
> If you're advocating for a senior, make sure home needs are attended to—yard work, house repair, and cleaning are all part of the treatment plan for any home owner. My mother's gardener and plumber have become advocates and members of her healing team.

Pay attention to important needs related to aging: hearing aids, eyeglasses, and adequate lighting, to name a few. Be sure that all necessary medications are available, and that there's a system for taking them as prescribed. Be aware of any chronic or acute problems that may exist beyond the primary diagnosis—these may require treatment, too. If the person you're advocating for is taking complementary medications or herbal preparations, check with the doctor to be sure that the combination won't cause complicating side effects.

Asking the Right Questions

To advocate well, you have to ask a lot of questions. You should constantly be asking the patient, "Do you have any questions? Is there anything I can do for you? How are you feeling? What's on your mind?" In some ways you're like a defense attorney, knowing the facts and probing for key important information so that your "defendant" is understood by the jury of health professionals and yourself.

If the answers you get are all negative—"No, I'm fine. I don't need anything. There are no problems"—don't accept them as the truth. Those are probably not honest answers. Children and mothers are especially prone to denying their feelings and needs in an attempt to make their families happy. Some overly cooperative people even put off dying until their loved ones leave the room. It's a fact that most deaths in the hospital occur in the wee hours of the morning, when family members and physicians aren't around.

So don't be dissuaded by assurances by your loved one that everything is fine and she has no needs—keep asking. Your questions will let her know that you really care and that you want to know how you can help. If you're advocating for an aging parent, be sure to let her know that she doesn't have to deny her problems to make her children happy.

It may sound like being an advocate is a lot of work, and in a sense it is. But don't be intimidated. If you have the right motive, and if you're giving your time and energy freely—out of compassion and true concern for someone who needs your help—then you'll be expressing the love that heals. Your only job is to help your loved one along the healing path she chooses. You don't have to know everything. In fact, an advocate who insists that he always knows what's right for someone else is so dangerous that we caution patients: *If you have an advocate who claims to know it all, then it's time to find a new one.*

❧

The relationship between an advocate and a patient can be deep and satisfying, and it may even end up being one of the blessings that comes from the illness. A young woman we helped sent us a poem in which she talks about a secret place, deep within each of us, where we go to get away to be alone and think things through. In this deep place, we find the essence of who we are and what we want to be. Now and then, someone comes along and discovers a way into that place of ours, and we may choose to allow them to share all that's stored there. When you advocate well, you may find that you've gone to that secret place and become a true friend to someone who needs you.

ى

CHAPTER 11

How to Be a Healing Visitor

You may never be called on to advocate for a loved one, but you probably will have occasion to visit someone you care about in the hospital. Does the thought of visiting make you uncomfortable? Do you worry that you won't know what to say or do when you have to spend time with someone who's confronted by a serious health problem? If you'd rather do just about *anything* than visit someone who's ill—a condition we call *visitaphobia*—then we have some good news. We can show you how to have relaxed and productive visits that are healing experiences for both you and the person you're visiting.

You may have good reasons for being anxious about spending time with someone who's ill. You may be scared about her condition or prospects, or her pain or suffering. You have no way of knowing what frame of mind she'll be in when you arrive. Or you may not have had pleasant visiting experiences in the past, and now you're bracing yourself for difficulties.

At the same time, your loved one may be having similar worries about the impending visit. She may feel that it's her responsibility to reassure you and to help deflect your anxiety or discomfort, especially if she's used to playing a caregiver role in the family.

Visiting should be as natural as breathing. But believe it or not, people take courses on how to do that, too! Why? Because they've forgotten the correct way to breathe—knowledge every baby possesses. In the same way, many of us have lost our natural ability to visit because we've forgotten how to be truly present in the moment—something children are experts at.

You can relearn everything you need to know about visiting by watching Uncle Chris Halvorsen, the large, swashbuckling, rough-and-tumble, fun-loving uncle in the 1948 film *I Remember Mama*. Rent the video—you'll love it and learn from it. Uncle Chris (played by Oscar Homolka) is the enemy of all pretentiousness and suffering. In one scene, he visits his nephew Arne, who's just had leg surgery. Uncle Chris sits at Arne's bedside, reading him a story. The boy quickly makes it clear that he doesn't want his uncle reading to him, then Arne screams in pain. Uncle Chris stops reading and begins singing in a deep baritone: "Ten thousand Swedes ran through the weeds at the Battle of Copenhagen, ten thousand Swedes ran through the weeds chasing one Norwegian!"

They both laugh, and then Arne moans in pain again and asks, "Uncle Chris, does it have to hurt like this?"

His uncle answers, "If you want to be well and not walk like Uncle Chris, then it does have to hurt for a little while." He suggests that if the boy doesn't think of his discomfort, then maybe he'll fall asleep. The boy groans again, and the uncle offers him a Norwegian swearword to say when the pain gets bad, and an "extra-strength" word to use if it gets worse. During the next wave of pain, Arne delightedly yells out the epithet and giggles with his uncle. Uncle Chris starts to belt out another tune, and Arne asks him to sing softer. He obliges, and Arne falls off to sleep. The scene ends with Uncle Chris—pleased and relieved—taking a sip from his whiskey flask.

That's Empowered Visiting 101 in a nutshell. Uncle Chris illustrates a lesson we taught in an earlier chapter: Pain is an essential part of life, and it protects us. But suffering is optional—it can be eliminated with the help of a visitor like Uncle Chris.

Let's rewind the tape and see how Uncle Chris helps his nephew heal. Right from the start, he's totally present. He sits rather than stands, so that he's eye-to-eye with Arne, and he begins checking out the boy's mind-set. He tests out one way of engaging him (reading aloud), and notices that this isn't what his nephew wants. Uncle Chris tries again, finding an activity that he and Arne can enjoy together: singing. When his nephew interrupts with shouts of pain, Uncle Chris acknowledges the boy's pain and offers a form of "distraction therapy"—in this case, cursing. When the waves of pain arrive, the boy is able to turn his attention to the swearwords he has learned. In addition to being fun, the swearing provides a sense of control—the boy now has something he can "do" about the pain.

(Distraction therapy, or "positive distraction," offers a very potent form of pain control and anxiety reduction—without the side effects of medication. It comes in many forms, from humor to visualization, and it's especially useful for children—but it also works well with adults: It's the principle behind the success of Bedscapes®, the healing tools we described earlier that use natural scenes and sounds to turn hospital cubicle curtains into pleasant environments.)

Yet to be a healing visitor, you don't need to memorize Uncle Chris's routine, nor do you need to figure out a clever way to take your loved one's mind off her ailment. In fact, visitors really don't need to do anything but be there and care. You may not know it, but the word *care* is related to the gothic word *kara,* which means "to grieve, express sorrow, or cry out with." So sometimes what a patient needs most isn't advice, reassurance, or distraction, but for you to join in her pain. You're not there to cure—you're there to visit, witness, and be present on the journey.

Before an Empowering Visit

If you want to relax and let things happen naturally, you may need to free yourself from the ghosts of "visits past," and forget the roles you and your loved one think you're supposed to play. Instead, take an optimistic approach to visiting, and focus on being both empowered and empowering—empowered, so that you can do everything you're capable of doing to help your loved one; and empowering, so that it will be easier for her to get herself the care she needs.

As an empowered visitor, know that *you* are the medicine because you're a carrier and channel of love, which is the most important element in healing. You already have everything you need to be a healing presence—so just allow yourself to be guided by your life experience and inner wisdom. This isn't a job for your head, it's a job for your heart.

Using your heart, you can assess the quality of care your loved one is receiving, and then, being empowered, you can do whatever feels necessary to assure that he or she gets the care that's needed. This is especially important if the patient is in a health-care facility, where you'll need to be able to see possibilities rather than limitations, solutions rather than problems, and breathing room and expansiveness rather than rules and regulations. Keep in mind that every encounter with another person is an opportunity for healing, and you'll see the professional health-care staff as fellow members of a healing team, not as adversaries.

We've come up with some coaching tips to make your visits as healing as possible, for both you and the patient. As we've noted in early chapters, you don't need to do everything we suggest here—the idea is to look at your options and follow the paths that are right for you and the person you're visiting. After all, empowered visitors know there's only one important question: "How does this help my loved one to heal?"

Before leaving for the hospital. Think of things you can bring that will help make your loved one's hospital room more nurturing, familiar, connected to his normal life, and more conducive to relaxation and play. You might bring pillows, comforters, family photos, paintings, or bulletin boards. You could bring hand lotion or the pleasant aroma of potpourri. Don't forget the always-essential comfort foods—any edibles that make your loved one feel cared for. (Be sure to ask the nursing staff if there are any dietary restrictions.) It's also a good idea to bring along something to occupy *your* time in case your loved one is resting when you arrive.

Check with someone who's visited recently and ask if your loved one has any practical or emotional needs you can fulfill. Maybe he needs a new Vital Sign, or maybe he'd like it if you offered to drive another one of his friends to the hospital with you.

If this is your first visit, you might want to check with the staff before you leave for the hospital. Call and ask for the nurses' station for the unit your loved one is in. Ask if it's appropriate for you to visit, and if you can call the patient directly. You may want to check to see if small children and pets are welcome—as we noted earlier, kids and animals are some of the most effective health-care providers we have. (There is one downside to calling ahead: The nurses we polled on this question were evenly split on the idea of being called before visits. The ones who didn't encourage pre-visit calls were concerned that they already have too little time for important patient-care tasks due to lack of staff. But these nurses still agreed that it's appropriate to call ahead if your loved one is in critical condition or is about to have a procedure done.)

It helps if you're able to talk to your loved one directly. That way, he's in control of his own time, he has an opportunity to tell you what he'd like you to bring, and he'll also get to enjoy the pleasant feeling of anticipating your visit. But this also gives him the chance to decline a visit if he doesn't want one. If he does decline, pay attention to what he says and use your intuition to figure out what he means. If he tells you not to visit, is that because he really doesn't want company, or is he trying to be nice and save you the trouble?

When you arrive at the hospital. This is a time for letting go and allowing your inner wisdom to inspire and guide you. Before you go to your loved one's unit, consider spending some time in the chapel, meditation space, or healing garden. Take a few minutes to let go of whatever else is going on in your life—your worries, concerns, obligations, and deadlines. Be present in the moment. You may want to try a brief visualization or prayer that focuses on the healing of your loved one. Do your best to witness his experience, and focus on what *you* would want if you were in his place.

When you arrive at your loved one's unit. Before going to the room, stop by the nurses' station and ask how the patient is doing. Most nurses we surveyed supported this step, but they noted that you might need to wait. Nurses are generally very busy and almost always have to stop doing something in order to attend to you. Remember, whether or not you have an explicit agreement with the nurses, you're all on the same healing team, and you all have the same goal: helping your loved one to heal. The first few times you stop by, you may feel like an interloper—and you may be treated as one. But watch this change as time passes and the staff becomes more familiar with you and aware that you're on the same side.

Begin by introducing yourself and asking if there's anything you need to know before your visit. The nurses may or may not answer this question—there may be confidentiality issues they need to respect, but they'll provide you with important information and insights if they're able to. Even if they can't offer you much, your question will remind them of the patient's needs. It's always good that people know your loved one has caring people looking after him.

Next, move to the unexpected: Ask the nurses how you can help *them* during your visit. Can you assist with feeding, giving fluids, escorting your loved one to the bathroom, or helping him to walk or exercise? Again, the first few times you ask, you may not get much response. But over time, these dedicated people will begin to trust you and to see you as a teammate who can provide some of the loving care they'd give if they had more time.

At the threshold of the room. Before you enter, pause and take a few easy breaths. Picture a chest or locker outside the door—this is the place to leave your judgments, worries, guilt, and blame. If you really need these items, you can retrieve them when you depart—but while you're visiting, leave them in the locker. Remind yourself that you're not responsible for your loved one's condition; you're here to do all you can, which is simply to offer a loving, caring presence. Too often our anger at the disease ends up directed at the patient; taking this moment gives you the opportunity to release that unhealthy anger.

Perhaps the best, most loving thing you'll be able to do in your visit is imagine your loved one as whole and vibrant. In your mind's eye, she's already healed. To only see her as sick or less than perfect is to make her more acutely and fearfully aware of her illness, and this impedes the healing process. You can offer a vision of her as whole. This isn't pretense or denial—it's loving visualization.

You have one last thing to do before entering: Forgive yourself, in advance, for anything you do that might later strike you as awkward or stupid. If you do something that you feel bad about during the visit, just say, "I'm sorry," and don't make excuses or blame someone else for your mistake.

Before you go in, remember: *You* are the medicine. Your presence is a gift. You're not there to do anything in particular; you're there to be present.

Now you're ready to enjoy a healing visit.

During an Empowering Visit

Entering the room. Knock first, even if the door is open or you hear people talking in the room, and wait for an answer. If you don't hear one, go to the nurses' station and ask someone to check with your loved one to see if you can visit. This isn't being overly formal; it's being respectful of your loved one's privacy and her ability to control her immediate environment. Such simple signs of respect are healing actions that serve as chicken soup for the psyche and megavitamins for the immune system.

When you're invited in, enter the room slowly and take in the scene. Assess the situation, taking cues from the patient and using all of your senses and your intuition. Ask your loved one if this is a good time to visit, or if she'd rather you came back later. If she feels guilty, she may think that this is your way of asking for permission not to visit. If she says that she'd rather you came back at another time, make sure that this is what she really wants. If it's a genuine request, then arrange a better time to return.

If it's a good time for a visit, ask her how long she'd like you to stay, or tell her to let you know when you should leave so she can rest. Again, many people feel guilty and say what they think you want to hear, so don't overdo it by asking for exact details. Just say, "If you get tired, let me know, or close your eyes and rest when you need to." It will be a much more relaxing visit for you both when it's clear that she really wants company and that she'll be able to end the visit easily if she needs to.

How long should visits last? The nurses we surveyed agreed that short, frequent visits are better than long, infrequent ones. Short ones don't tire the patient, and when you come more often, it gives her the chance to anticipate seeing people, getting news, and staying connected to family and community. Remember that we're talking about visits—not about the occasions where you might need to tend to a loved one virtually around the clock.

You've probably heard the injunction to physicians: "Do no harm." This applies to you, the visitor, as well. Your first order of business is to do no harm. As long as you relax, listen, observe, and pay attention during your visit, you'll succeed.

The listening part is especially important. We all need someone who will hear what we have to say. Helen Keller knew the value of listening—she said that deafness is darker by far than blindness. When you visit, be present and lend your ear. If you listen to your loved one, no matter what she has to say, she'll thank you for your help. If you listen a little, and then tell her what she should do, she probably won't thank you, because you'll be more of a problem than a helper. People who are ill need to make sense of what's going on in their lives and the choices they have to make about their care. The best way to help your loved one make choices is to listen to her discuss them.

We offer just three fundamentals to guide empowered and empowering visitors:

- Trust your own inner wisdom.

- Trust in the power of love to inform and guide you.

- Trust in the power of healthy, healing humor.

Dayle Friedman, a rabbi who trains rabbis and chaplains to be present with those who are ill or suffering, makes it easy to remember how to conduct yourself as a visitor. She suggests three simple ground rules for bedside visiting: (1) Sit down, (2) shut up, and (3) connect. Here's how Rabbi Friedman's guidelines can help you become an empowering visitor.

Sit down. The title of a meditation book by Sylvia Boorstein tells you how to start your visit: *Don't Just Do Something, Sit There!* This is a variation on a piece of advice that an acting coach once offered his students, who were too busy "acting" to ever get around to just "being" in their roles: "Don't just do something, stand there!" Sitting puts you and your loved one at the same eye level and, in a broader sense, on the same plane. As we learned from Uncle Chris, this simple act helps set the tone for a more relaxed, healing visit.

Shut up. Don't feel you have to say anything. Again, remember the value of simply being present. Your quiet sitting may be the beginning of a silent visit, or the visit may go on to involve a lot of talk. But if you begin by shutting up, then you'll have a better chance of finding out what kind of visit will serve your loved one best.

She may be having a bad day and may be in poor spirits. She could be angry, scared, in pain, depressed, or confused from medications. The best strategy for this visit might be a quiet, loving presence, where you simply witness how she's feeling. Don't deny her feelings or try to fix what she's going through. You're a witness, not a therapist. If you're willing and able to listen, let your loved one know that you're open to hearing anything she has to say. She may or may not take you up on this offer. The choice is hers, and just having the option of unburdening herself may be a comfort in itself. Alternately, you may find that the medicine of the day is laughing, singing, or engaging in physical activity such as therapeutic physical exercises.

Connect. The first step in connecting, Rabbi Friedman suggests, is remembering *why* you're visiting. You're there with your loved one because you care enough to be present during this difficult time. You want to help in the healing process, and your loving connection is important. Although being there is the most important thing you do, you can also perform simple comforting tasks to soothe her. Does she need the headboard light turned off or put in the indirect (aiming up) position? Does her bedding need to be straightened out? Pillows fluffed? Does she need the elevation of the bed adjusted or the cubicle curtain repositioned? Do the flowers need fresh water? Are her personal items within easy reach? If she's unconscious or unable to communicate easily, you can assess the situation yourself and take care of these comforting tasks.

Helping your loved one with these simple tasks does more than make her comfortable—it also helps her feel more self-sufficient and in control. Studies have shown that people who feel a greater sense of control over their immediate environment tend to have stronger immune systems. Your loved one needs to be able to manipulate her immediate environment, whether she's in a health-care facility or convalescing at home. Every task she can do for herself promotes her sense of control and boosts her immune system. A feeling of dependency can lead to a downward spiral, while self-sufficiency and a sense of control lead to vitality and energy. You can make a big difference in your loved one's life during this difficult time by talking with her about her needs and making sure that the items she wants are within reach.

Visiting Elderly Friends and Relatives

All the visiting tips we've mentioned apply when you visit your elderly friends and relatives. Again, the major gift you bring is yourself, your presence and your love. The key is love—everything else, as they say, is commentary.

Before visiting an older patient, you can go through the same preparations we've already described. When you arrive, be sure to knock before entering, even if it's your father who's the patient. If there's no answer, you might ask a nurse to see if he's open to a visit. Again, this isn't silly protocol—it's a way of supporting your dad's sense of control. For the same reason, begin the visit by asking him how long he'd like you to stay. Remember that extended visits can be tiring, and that briefer, more frequent visits are generally better.

When you're visiting parents, it can be especially difficult to remember that you're not there to fix them. You can't make everything right and you can't create and maintain the ultimate healing environment for them. Your dad's healing journey is his, not yours. You can't change what he's going through and the circumstances he finds himself in. You're not responsible for his illness—if you believe you are, then you need to find a way to let go of that belief. Feeling responsible for your dad's problems won't help him, and it won't help you, either. It's natural to feel sad about what he's going through, but if you take on guilt, too, you won't be able to be helpful.

If you want to help your father, do everything you can to make sure he's comfortable. Let him know that you love him. Help him feel safe, secure, and confident that his wishes will be respected.

Try to witness his experience by putting yourself in his place and asking yourself what decisions you'd make if you were in his shoes—remember, these may be different than the choices you'd make as the grown child or caregiver. Encourage him to participate in discussions about medications, treatments, operations, diet, or exercise, but don't bully him into taking on a more active role than he chooses. His life experience isn't yours, and he may need to have unquestioning faith in his doctor. It's his life, and he gets to choose how much he wants to be in charge of his care and how much information he needs.

No matter how great your love for your father is, or what you think is the best for him, you don't get to choose which healing paths are right for him. This isn't a time to preach about why he must change his ways. If you do that, you're apt to make him feel like a failure, and you can end up doing more harm than good.

We know that it's hard to see someone you love doing things that can cause him harm or will fail to help him. When you think about this, though, you may find something familiar and funny about the situation: Didn't our moms and dads have the same experience in the years they were parenting us—in some cases well into our so-called adult years? How open were we to their wisdom? Our job now is to care for them and help them love themselves. Anything else we offer, such as advice on treatments or lifestyle choices, they'll either accept or reject, depending on what seems right to them.

Let's not forget that our elders have been around longer than we have, so a visit is also an opportunity to receive wisdom—it's an opportunity for a "senior moment." We're not talking about forgetfulness—which is another matter altogether. (Most of us have brief episodes of forgetfulness that are nothing more than our souls crying out for a moment of respite from the psychic overload of daily life. The lapses elders suffer from are often due to the opposite problem—psychic *under*load—and a lack of engaged, loving contact with other people.) When *we* talk about "senior moments," we're referring to those times when our elders share their insights with us. You can increase the likelihood of one of these positive moments by making your parent feel comfortable, relaxed, and respected. It also helps if you share your problems and ask her to give you some of her hard-earned wisdom. She'll feel useful, and you'll be better off.

> **Yosaif:** I had a healing breakthrough with my father when I asked what I could do to make it easier for him to relate to me. He immediately replied, "Ask my advice when it has a chance of making a difference in what you do."

> **Bernie:** My 94-year-old mother gave her granddaughter advice about the correct time to have another baby. When my mom is advising younger generations, she forgets her multiple afflictions. Her good senior moments turn out to be a beneficial exchange: The family gains her wisdom, and she's healed by distraction therapy.

We miss out on these experiences when we take on the inappropriate role of parenting our parents. It's even worse if we treat them as infants and talk about them in their presence. There may be a time in your life when you must care for your parents, but this isn't a role reversal. Remember, to your mother and father, you're still the child, despite your age or the responsibility you take on; and they're still the parents, even if the care they need now seems similar to what a child might need.

When you visit an elder, you're often doing it for his or her benefit, but in these senior moments there are plenty of opportunities for reciprocity.

> **Yosaif:** My wife serves as a chaplain and a pastoral counselor at nursing homes and hospitals. Sometimes

during a visit with an elder, she'll ask for a blessing. Most patients are delighted to oblige, and they usually offer blessings full of wisdom.

Many of us have highly charged relations with our parents. If your relationship with your mother or father is difficult, you can begin to heal it now. Start by acting as if you feel the way you'd like to. Act as if you love your parents right now, and keep it up until you do. Remember that love is blind to faults.

When an aging parent is ill, you have the opportunity to reconnect, heal, or complete your relationship. This important topic is beyond the scope of this book, but there are now abundant sources you can find in your local bookstore to guide you in this healing work. Keep your eye out for the word *forgiveness*. As the saying goes, *If not now, when?*

The path to being an empowered and empowering visitor is straightforward: Relax, be present, and take your cues from your loved one. See healing possibilities instead of barriers, and have something mutually rewarding to do—whether it's being quiet together or sharing a therapeutic activity.

We all want the things we do to have meaning. We want to experience life fully, to live as if every moment is as fresh as our first and as precious as our last. The hours we spend visiting loved ones who are convalescing can be deeply satisfying and full of meaning. Let them be among the most rewarding times we've ever spent together.

Now that you're prepared to visit your loved one, there's one more person who needs some healing attention: you. In the next chapter, we'll talk about how you can see to it that your own needs are met while you're helping your loved one to heal.

CHAPTER 12

Healing for the Caregiver

This chapter is geared toward anyone who's helping somebody to heal. You may be reading this because a loved one has asked you to sign on as a healing teammate, or perhaps you've taken on the important job of being an advocate for someone you care about. Or maybe you picked up this book because you're a professional caregiver—a doctor, nurse, or therapist. Whoever you are, however you came to be a caregiver, we want to help you think about your own healing.

When we talk about healing, we're not talking about the condition of your body as much as we're referring to the condition of your life. The words *heal* and *holy* are both derived from the same Old English word that meant "to make whole." When you realize what healing is, you can see how a person with an incurable physical problem can be healed and whole—as well as holy. You can also see that you, a caregiver who isn't physically ill, still need to pay attention to your own wholeness, even while you help someone else.

We get lots of letters and e-mails from people who are experiencing illness in their family and want to share their pain and wounds, and we often hear from medical professionals as well.

One doctor recently wrote to tell us about his experience with his father's illness. "For the first time, I'm experiencing illness from a patient's perspective," the doctor wrote. "How can we as a family be more effective in relieving the agony and anguish my father must be experiencing? Are there programs you can offer to enhance his chance of recovery?"

Those are good questions, but before we answer them, we want to note one irony: The doctor who wrote us is probably suffering more than most nonphysicians would be in his situation. Not only does medical training *not* help him deal with illness in his own family, it's likely to leave him worse off.

> **Bernie:** You'd that think a medical education would help prepare you for the feelings you experience when someone you care about is ill, but the truth is that most medical schools ignore emotions and train you to expect the worst. I know. As I've described in earlier books, my medical training didn't prepare me at all for how I'd feel about illness. I was lost until my patients began to teach me all the important things medical schools ignore.
>
> I began to learn about healing in 1977, around the time I first shaved my head. At the time, this was totally unfashionable, and it served as a sign that I was a troubled human being. But as soon as I did it, everyone at the hospital began sharing their problems with me. Why? Because it was obvious that I was wounded, and people assumed— correctly—that someone wounded would be better able to understand their pain.
>
> When people ask me, "How are you?" I sometimes answer, "Depressed. I'm out of my medication, my doctor is away, and I can't renew my prescription." Three-quarters of the people I run into will respond, "I know how you feel." Then they'll share information about their lives, reveal their wounds, and offer me their medications! The few people who don't respond by sharing their problems

are generally those who are healed, and they give me love to help me on my journey.

If you don't believe this, go out into the world limping and using a cane, and watch how people respond to you.

Preparing to Be a Caregiver

So how does one become an instant caregiver with no advance warning or training? How do you take on the job while keeping your life reasonably balanced and as whole as possible? How do you keep your spirits up for the long haul without becoming exhausted—emotionally, physically, and spiritually?

We wouldn't have to ask these questions if we trained our children and families to prepare for the difficulties that inevitably lie ahead for all of us. To prepare, we need to discuss what we want, what's important to us, and what we'll do when problems arise. Life is a school: We can use the events that occur every day in our lives to discuss our needs and develop strategies for coping with problems. We don't have to leave this to last-minute guesswork. When you talk things over, the best thing you can do is listen to each other. The person sharing her fears usually realizes for herself where the solution lies, because describing the problem clarifies the issues and leads directly to solutions.

If you're put in a position where you must become a caregiver instantly, know that you can do it—even without having been trained. Just allow yourself to be guided by your feelings and those of the person you're caring for. The same rules apply to you both: The caregiving shouldn't drain you or deplete you, and you don't have to sacrifice yourself.

As we often point out, you can learn about healing relationships from watching animals. They don't ask questions—they make noise to get attention, display their emotions, and move or reach out to get what they want. A veterinarian once wrote to us about how observing her animal patients helped her through her mastectomy: "I can amputate half of a jaw or a leg, and the animals will awaken and lick their owner's faces," she observed. "They're here to love and be loved—and to teach us a few things about life."

The veterinarian is right. Animals know that they're whole no matter what their physical condition is. We humans have yet to achieve that awareness. The Bible tells us in many places that animals are our teachers, and God didn't have to give them any instructions because they're already complete. We can learn from their examples if we put aside our fear of paying attention to our feelings and following our intuition.

As a caregiver, you're responsible for making sure that your own needs are met, too. Get some caregivers of your own, and seek help from a therapist or support group if you need it. Set limits on what you do so that you don't burn out, and maintain your own health by doing the same things that you're urging the person in your care to do: meditate, practice yoga, exercise, eat well, get a massage, listen to music, and enjoy pleasant aromas. This will really help, because when you meditate or exercise, your body produces its own antidepressants. Look back at the earlier chapters that provide tips for healing activities and environments—most of the tips we provided for patients are appropriate for you, too.

Don't forget to take a break or Sabbath time. Get others to fill in for you so that you won't feel guilty taking time for yourself. But tell the patient why you're taking a break. Don't leave it to his imagination—he may come up with destructive thoughts and negative reasons for your absence if you don't explain why you're temporarily unavailable.

Bernie: I used to share my phone number with some patients even when I was on vacation. I didn't feel guilty and they rarely called—just knowing I was available was usually enough.

Let go of solving all the world's problems. You are the caregiver, not the *cure*giver. Maintain your life and your routines, and continue doing the things you enjoy. Keep a journal and educate yourself about your needs while you discover the needs of the person you're caring for. These activities restore you so that you can be a healing presence. Take time to take care of yourself and you'll have more energy to help others.

Doctors As Caregivers

The word *doctor* is derived from a Latin word that means "teacher" or "to teach." Doctors teach healing best when they're in the process of becoming more whole themselves—that's the reason for the old saying, "Physician, heal thyself." To be an effective healer, a physician has to be a native, not a tourist, in the land of the wounded. If she doesn't acknowledge her own wounds and isn't in the process of healing, then she'll remain a visitor who can only treat and prescribe. She can't heal, because she doesn't deal with the patient's experience and doesn't relieve suffering.

We can all be healers if we have the courage to share our pain. We can't fix everything, but we can help heal everyone. This is the message for the doctor at the beginning of this chapter who wrote for advice on his father's illness: There's more to treat than diseases and symptoms. When professional caregivers realize that they can focus their attention on the entire person and not just his illness, they feel empowered and useful. It's never too late for a doctor to care, no matter how far a disease has progressed or how ill a patient is. Even after a patient dies, there are family members and friends who still need care—and the doctor will need it, too.

Remember the Basics of Healing

You heal your life the same way you help others heal theirs—with love and humor. These are the keys to creating a state of wholeness and holiness. When you love and laugh, you're a child again—free of afflictions. You may feel as if you're in a trance, free of bodily ailments and concerns. You'll know that you're in a state of healing and atonement—or *at-one-ment*—with creation when you love and laugh enough to lose track of time.

Remember that only love is immortal. We're all going to die, and most of us are going to be ill at some point. But we can still be well, because wellness isn't just a question of what's happening in our bodies, but in our minds and spirits as well. We know many people who have afflictions that can never be cured but who are quite well because they're at peace with others, themselves, and their lives.

We can learn about healing by watching how animals remain complete all their lives. They live in harmony with their creator—they don't whine or make excuses, they never blame anyone for anything, and they never worry that their disease is related to their guilt or shame.

We read in the Bible that God looked at creation and called it *good*. This is a mistranslation. The word should read "complete," or "whole." By the same token, our job as humans is to find completion within ourselves. Our teachers are our afflictions—through them, we can discover the path toward wholeness, holiness, and wellness.

Whether you're giving care as a visitor, advocate, physician, or nurse, remember that it's about more than just curing diseases. Know that you don't fail or lose when someone dies despite your therapy and your prayers. Whenever you're able to help an afflicted person feel whole, you're being a successful caregiver.

If you insist on seeing disease and death as failures, you put yourself in an unhealthy position where it's almost impossible to get close to patients and truly care for them. Many caregivers end up suffering from post-traumatic stress disorder because they don't have a time or place to discuss how they feel about the illnesses they encounter and the losses they experience. Their pain remains within, where it takes its physical and emotional toll.

Remember the teaching we mentioned earlier in this book: If you don't bring forth what's within you, it will destroy you. If you *do* bring forth what's within you, it will save you. If you keep your feelings imprisoned, they can literally break your heart. If you allow yourself to become aware of your feelings, and respond to them, you can stay healthy. Take the time to keep a journal of your dreams and feelings, practice daily prayer or meditation, and attend group meetings to discuss your emotions. While you're doing this, take a look at the deeper, more significant reasons why you chose to be a caregiver.

We happen to be outside advisors to the Board of Directors of Heaven, and we can tell you that vegetarians, meditators, joggers, and the faithful all die. Some of them are quite bitter about dying after all the time and effort they put into trying to live forever. So don't waste your life trying to avoid death. Try instead to live fully, following your own unique and authentic path, and in the process you'll live the longest, fullest life possible for you. As it says in the Bible, "He who seeks to keep his life will lose it, and whoever loses his life will preserve it," (Luke 17:33).

We've seen many people recover from life-threatening illnesses when they learned that they had only a short time left to live. At the moment they were told that they were going to die, they began to live their true lives, following what was in their hearts. As a result, some of these people felt so good that they didn't die from their affliction.

If you choose to become a caregiver, then make sure that you're doing it for the right reasons. Do it because it's the right path for you, not because you feel guilty or someone else wants you to do it. Ask yourself, "What do I have to offer those I can't cure?"

So what should the doctor tell his father who is ill with cancer? We don't think his words will heal his dad's cancer, no matter how great they might be. After all, what do you say to give a quadriplegic man the will to live? Since you can walk, you don't know what he's experiencing. You're a tourist and not a native, so rather than preach, bring the natives together in groups and let them share their experiences to guide, support, and heal each other.

Denying our mortality is hard work and a prescription for illness. We're healthier when we accept that we'll all eventually die. Then we can begin to live our lives, expressing our love in our own unique ways and registering our righteous indignation when we're not treated with respect. When we accept our mortality, we can learn to play, express our needs and feelings, make decisions, say no to things we don't want to do, and use our pain to redirect our lives.

We believe that everyone is a child of God, precious in the Creator's sight. We think that God created a world in which difficulties exist so that we could have the experience of being caregivers and co-creators. Too often we see people bring flowers to the grave and weep at the funeral of a loved one, after having missed the chance to show up with bouquets and tears of empathy while the person they cared about was still alive. All human beings are here to show compassion to the living, to love and to create a Garden of Eden by our choices and our actions. When we do what we're here for—caring for ourselves and each other—we become ageless and free from all afflictions.

Can you picture Mother Teresa complaining about how difficult it is to be a caregiver? Sure, she looked tired, but we never heard her gripe—and we can't imagine her being burned out. What did she know that the doctor at the beginning of this chapter didn't know? Mother Teresa knew that we as caregivers need to live out the wisdom that's in our hearts. Then we're not working—we're creating and experiencing the wholeness that our Creator intended for us. The doctor who wrote with questions about how to care for his father was used to being guided by his head. We're not criticizing him—he cared about his father and was in pain, and he was asking the right questions. He only needed to know what we all need to discover: The answers to our questions about health and healing are in our hearts.

If you can pay attention to your intuition, follow your heart wisdom, and take time for your own healing, then you're ready to care for others. In Part III ("Healing Ways"), you'll find more tips on healing, including detailed instructions on massage, bedside yoga, and other activities that can help you and your loved ones to heal.

꒜

PART III

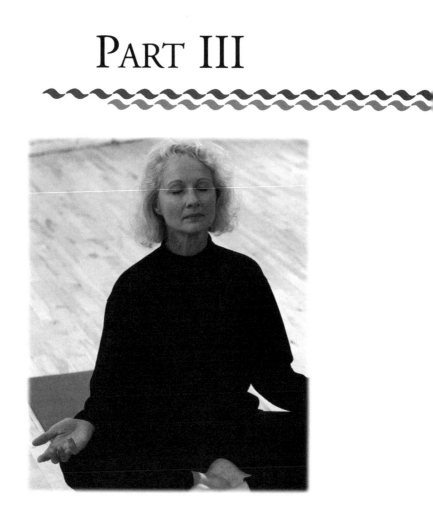

Healing Ways

CHAPTER 13

Activities That Heal

*Tips for Patients: Turning Bedside Visits
into Healing Encounters*

During the course of your treatment, you may go through many conflicting feelings. You may feel a sense of loss, yet at the same time experience a sense of relief and release. Your body might register anger at having been invaded by surgery, chemotherapy, or radiation, even while you're amazed and grateful that the treatment eliminated a diseased part. On a spiritual level, it's likely that you've endured the medical procedures you've gone through as a form of separation, brokenness, or a disruption of wholeness.

But your wholeness doesn't depend on an inventory of body parts—it's a condition of *being*. So while the "healing ways" listed in this chapter are intended to promote physical healing and rehabilitation, they'll also help you adjust to new limitations and find new ways of living with them—either temporarily or longer term. (We do mean *living* with limitations, not just gritting your teeth and suffering from them.) Our healing ways are physical exercises that can help you improve your health and level of comfort, resolve your conflicted emotions, and move toward emotional wholeness.

The assistance of a physical therapist can work wonders for patients, but there's so much demand for their time in the hospital that they won't be able to meet all of your needs for exercise. Wherever you may be convalescing, there are some simple things you can do—alone or with a companion—that will feel good and help you to heal. When you offer your family and visitors the opportunity to join you in these activities, you'll open up a whole new range of possibilities for your bedside encounters. Healing benefits will flow in both directions. After you've found an activity that works for you, you can extend those benefits by doing it when you're alone as well.

You can get yourself on a path to wholeness with the healing ways we describe in this book: bedside yoga, walking and wheelchairing, and massage. Bedside-yoga exercises are a gentle antidote to the kind of deterioration that can occur in your body when you're immobile, and they get you into a healing frame of mind by reminding you what it feels like to be alive and vibrant. They can also help you lovingly reconnect with your body after medical treatment. Walking and wheelchairing will make getting up and about more interesting, engaging, and fun. And the massage instruction will guide your companion to help you feel comforted and relaxed.

We suggest that you ask your physician, nurse, and physical therapist for advice on which activities are most appropriate right now, and what pace or intensity they recommend. Then check back periodically to see what changes they may advise you to make as your condition evolves. But before choosing an exercise, read it through and see if your intuition tells you that it's right for you.

Before you begin, you may want to try talking to your body— or to a specific part that's been the site of trauma. Words have power, which is why techniques such as guided visualization are so effective. But this power is a double-edged sword, and just as we can give our bodies "love" and "live" messages, we often unconsciously say things to ourselves that are much less kind. Have you ever heard people refer to their "bad back" or say that their neck is "killing" them? Imagine if instead they simply said, "My back is in distress; it could use some TLC." What difference do you think it would make in how they felt over time? The next time you feel uncomfortable, try it—and be prepared for nice things to happen. Love your body—especially the part that has the disease—and you'll heal more quickly.

Bedside yoga and massage are ways of giving love to your body. They're less about technique and more about exploration, so as you begin an exercise, be easy and gentle with yourself, and experience it sensually—pay attention to how it feels and what your inner sense tells you. You're beginning to reconnect with that part of your body, so don't force anything; simply be aware.

Once you get going, you and your healing team can find an abundance of other resources in your local library or bookstore, or on the Internet. These may include guided healing meditations and visualizations that we have developed (available on the ECaP Website: **www.ecap-online.org**).

If you spend time engaged in healing activities while you're in the hospital, you won't fall into the role of submissive, suffering patient. Instead, you'll take control of your space and time and create experiences that contribute to your meaningful existence. You'll have the power to live and grow. Your Vital Signs, your visits with loved ones, and the activities you do on your own will keep you on a healing path, and soon you'll be ready to begin thinking about your next challenge: how to continue the healing process after you leave the hospital. Once you know what you'd like to do, and you and your companion have the tools to do it with, all you need to do is post a "Healing in Progress—Please Do Not Disturb" sign on your door or closed cubicle curtain. Time is of the essence here, so the sooner you get started, the better off you'll be. As the advertising slogan says: "Just do it!"

Tips for Families, Beside Companions, and Visitors

We know that you don't need anyone to coach you or instruct you in lovingly reaching out and touching your loved one—holding her hand, putting a warm or cool washcloth on her forehead, or giving her a hug. The healing ways we present here are meant to extend and enhance what you already do naturally.

Yosaif: My excitement about the healing potential of these exercises came from my experience of doing "bedside ballet" with my mother-in-law shortly after she suffered a stroke. As I mentioned earlier, my wife, Tsurah, and I believe that we were able to help her regain a significant amount of body mobility and vitality over the next few years by simply moving her arms and legs for her when she was unable to.

My last visit with my 85-year-old mother was also an inspiration. She was drooped over in a wheelchair after experiencing multiple strokes. Only months before, she had a great spring in her step, and at the drop of a hat she'd do a jitterbug or sing from a seemingly limitless repertoire of songs. I asked her how she felt about her situation. She roused herself and exclaimed, "It stinks!" and fell back into the slumped position. The situation *did* stink—she was tired of her body and ready to leave it very soon.

But in the meantime, I wanted her to feel my loving and caring. So I got some body lotion from the nursing staff and massaged my mother's hands and shoulders. I found massaging her hands to be an especially intimate experience. Even though I'm a physically affectionate person and I do a lot of hugging, I hadn't experienced my mother's hands close up since I was a young child. After massaging her hands for a few minutes, I brought her back to her room. That was the last time I saw my mother alive—a very sad time, but a very poignant experience of connecting.

You can have similarly intimate experiences if you use your heart and intuition to guide you in what you already do naturally.

Healing ways provide avenues to being lovingly engaged—they're not ways of escaping from connection by making yourself busy. Don't force healing ways; sometimes your loved one simply wants to enjoy your company and do nothing else but hang out together. The choices are up to you and the person in your care. Take the lead from him. When you try things out, you'll quickly get a sense of what's appropriate. The activities should feel comfortable and engaging for you as well as your loved one.

We recommend that you consult with your loved one's attending nurse, physician, physical therapist, or other healing professional about the appropriateness, timing, and intensity of any particular activity. You're all on the same healing team.

Remember the advice we offered in Chapter 11: Relax, forgive yourself for making mistakes, have fun, and trust your inner wisdom. Most of all, keep in mind that these activities are about healing *possibilities,* not limitations. You and your loved one will discover together what those opportunities are for you.

Bedside Yoga

A few general guidelines:

- Read through each exercise first to see if it feels right for you.

- Check with your medical team to see if the exercise you've selected is appropriate, and if so, what level of pacing and intensity is recommended.

• Be gentle and loving with yourself—remember, this isn't a performance.

Belly Breathing Exercise

Position: In bed

Benefits: Breathing can help you relax, relieve tension and stress, lessen or eliminate your pain, and connect with your spirit. It's an easy way to turn the time you spend waiting—for your physician, for test results, and so forth—into healing time.

Don't make "work" out of this. If you simply close your eyes, breathe easily, and pay attention to your breath, then you can get all the benefits described above. The following exercise can enhance your experience. Remember, it's not about rigidly adhering to a technique—it's about exploration.

Instructions:

1. On your bed, rest on your back with your legs bent. Separate your feet 16 to 18 inches apart and let your knees rest against one another. Place your hands gently on your belly, with your fingertips touching.

2. Breathe in through your nose and allow your belly to fill with air (expanding like a balloon). As you do this, feel your fingertips separating. As you exhale, be aware of your navel moving back toward your spine and your fingertips moving toward one another.

3. As you continue to breathe in this manner, try to keep your chest as still as possible, and allow your breath and movement to come from your belly. With each inhalation, gently feel your whole being expand. With each exhalation, release and relax more and more deeply.

4. Allow each breath to guide you on a journey inward so that you may connect with the stillness deep within you. Feel each inhalation arise out of this stillness and each exhalation dissolve back into it. Within this quiet place, feel the radiant inner peace and joy that is your birthright. Allow tension, fear, and anxiety to melt away in one irreversible stream as you exhale, and let peace fill your body, mind, and heart. As you inhale, feel your whole being radiating and reflecting tranquility as you relax even more deeply.

Shared Breathing Exercise

Position: In bed or in a chair

Benefits: This is an especially nice way to be present with someone you care about and who cares about you. Breathing together is a wonderful way to be connected.

Note to family and other team members: This activity has value whether your loved one is fully conscious, asleep, unconscious, or even comatose.

Instructions:

1. If possible, sit in chairs face-to-face with one another. If that's not possible, the patient can rest in bed in whatever position is comfortable.

2. The patient can close her eyes if that's comfortable. Begin to tune in to her breath. If you can hear her breathe, then follow her rhythm—breathing in when she inhales and breathing out when she exhales. If you can't hear her, then watch as her chest rises and falls, and begin to breathe with her.

3. Once you're in sync, close your eyes and simply breathe together. Allow yourself to relax more deeply with each exhalation.

4. Imagine that there's just one breath—allow any bound-
    aries between the two of you to melt away. Feel the deep
    connection to each other as you share this sacred moment.
    After breathing together for a few minutes, slowly open
    your eyes. If it's comfortable for you, you can bring your
    hands into a prayer position in front of your heart and
    bow to each other.

Leg Slides

Position: In bed
Benefits: This exercise improves the flexibility of your legs and
groin area.

Instructions:

1. Lie comfortably on your back. Keeping your legs togeth-
    er, stretch them out in front of you on the bed. Your legs
    should be straight, but your joints should be relaxed and
    not rigid. Let your arms rest gently at your side.

2. Take a deep breath in and hold it for a count of four.
    Exhale slowly as you mentally count to four. (You'll count
    to four each time you inhale or exhale during this exer-
    cise.) Inhale again, and this time, as you exhale, slide your
    right leg out to the right as far as you comfortably can,
    while keeping your left leg still. Don't arch your back.

3. Slowly inhale, bringing your right leg back in to its origi-
    nal position. Breathe out. Breathe in, and with the next
    exhale, slowly stretch your left leg out along the bed and
    to the left—as far as you comfortably can—and keep your
    right leg still. As you breathe in, bring your left leg back in
    to meet your right leg.

4. Repeat four times for each leg.

Shoulder Stretches

Position: Seated, either in bed or on a chair
Benefits: Improves circulation and range of motion and releases tension and tightness in your shoulders, neck, upper back, and chest.

Instructions:
1. Inhale and shrug both shoulders up toward your ears. Exhale and gently and firmly press both shoulders down. Repeat four times.

2. Inhale and bring your shoulders up toward your ears. As you exhale, roll your shoulders back, down, and then forward. Continue rolling your shoulders four times and then change directions.

Spine Flexes and Extensions

Position: Seated, on the edge of a bed or in a chair
Benefits: Warms, flexes, and extends the spine; energizes the intervertebral disks and spinal cord; opens the chest and gently stretches the back; and relieves tension in the area between the shoulder blades.

Instructions:
1. Sit on the edge of your bed or front edge of a chair with your arms out to your sides, palms facing up. Press your sitz bones (*ischial tuberosities,* the "sitting bones" at the base of your pelvis) down. At the same time, begin to bring your arms slightly back—keeping them straight until you feel your shoulder blades moving inward. Keep

your shoulders gently pressing downward away from your ears. Lift your chest and look slightly up.

2. Exhale and flex (round) your spine, one vertebra at a time, as you roll back onto your tailbone. Bring your arms forward and give yourself a hug, bringing your chin toward your chest.

3. Repeat six times, alternately flexing and extending your spine. Imagine yourself as a sea anemone opening and closing.

Walking and Wheelchairing

These days hospital staff members try to get patients out of bed, up on their feet, and walking as soon as possible. Why? Because the sooner a patient is up and about, the sooner she's healed enough to go home and get on with the next stages of recuperation and rehabilitation.

So why not fill these ventures with fun and discovery? Why not have frolics, escapades, or walking meditations? Here are a few suggestions for what to do when you're first able to get up and about, walking (with or without personal assistance or a support device) and wheelchairing:

- Make people smile. See if it works like yawning, which can be contagious. If you can't make them grin, then make them yawn!

- Stop by and see someone in another room who doesn't seem to have any visitors. Check with the nurses about who it might be best to visit.

- Do some "grateful watching." Observe a maintenance person doing his duties with an eye of appreciation. You can do it from afar, or you can do it up close and tell the person how you value the service he's doing.

- Do a gratefulness walk (or wheelchairing). Do laps around the corridors, and with each pass, think about one thing you're grateful for in your life. This is actually a kind of walking meditation. You may be surprised to discover how many blessings you have—and the serenity you can experience by doing this meditation.

Massage: The Healing Power of Touch

It's important to check with the health-care staff about the appropriateness of massage for your loved one at this time. Ask also for any particular guidelines or cautions, and continually check with your loved one as to how the massage feels. Wash your hands before and after.

Foot Massage

Position: In bed or seated. (If your loved one is in a chair, then hold his foot on your lap and be sure that his knee joint is relaxed, not rigid. If he's lying down, position yourself at his feet, facing his head. This massage can be done on bare feet or with socks on.)

Benefits: Improves circulation, increases flexibility, and provides healing contact for you and your loved one.

Instructions:
1. Grasp your loved one's foot gently using both hands, with your thumbs on the bottom of the foot and your fingers on top. Starting at the base of the toes and moving toward the heel, rub the sole of the foot with both thumbs. You

can make small circles, go back and forth, move up and down, or do all of the above. Find out which combinations feel good to you and your loved one.

2. With your hands in the starting position, use both thumbs to press into the sole of your loved one's foot. Begin gently, under the big toe. Press points along a line from the big toe to the heel, then return to the second toe and repeat the procedure with each of the other toes in turn. You can then go back to the big toe and repeat the entire exercise, pressing more deeply this time. Press as deeply as is comfortable for you and your loved one. Do this step several times.

3. Taking the heel in one hand and grasping just below the toes with the other, gently rotate the foot, first clockwise several times, then counterclockwise the same number of times.

4. With one hand supporting the heel and your other hand with the palm on the ball of the foot and fingers over the top of the toes, push the top of the foot up gently toward the knee. Push only as far as is comfortable for your loved one. On stretches like this, breathe in sync with your loved one.

5. Place your hands on each side of the heel just below the ankle, with the fingers pointing toward the head. Rub the heel lightly and briskly, moving the hands back and forth in opposite directions.

Hand Massage

Position: Seated or lying down

Instructions:

1. Cradle your loved one's hand, palm facing down, in both of your hands. Your fingers should be touching her palm, and your thumbs should reach around to the top of her hand. Rub the top of her hand with back-and-forth movements of your thumbs. Massage the entire area several times. Then, gently bend the wrist down as far as it will comfortably go once or twice. Do this for both hands.

2. Grasp the little finger with one hand while supporting the hand with your other hand. Beginning at the base of that finger, gently twist back and forth above each knuckle to massage the soft tissue there. Repeat on all fingers and thumbs.

3. Turn the hand palm up and grasp with both of your hands, your thumbs touching her palms and your fingers below. Use your thumbs to massage the entire palm, using circular and back-and-forth motions. Cover the area several times.

❈

Bernie's Resource List

In general, I shy away from reading lists. There are so many books available on the subject of health, healing, and self-empowerment that it would take a volume to list them all. If you have the inspiration and want the information, you can go to any good bookstore and ask for help finding self-help texts. At the front of this book, you can find a list of other titles I've written, as well as available audiotapes and videos. (Some of my earlier books include bibliographies with resources.)

If you're reading this because a loved one is ill, you can help him help himself. Present him with the resources mentioned here, and then step back. Listen to him, and then read everything for yourself so that you're ready to support him.

Medical journals are very specialized and limited, so you have to reach beyond them for information. So for both skeptics and believers, I recommend starting with books that helped me personally wake up and know I was on the right track: Among them are Lawrence LeShan's *You Can Fight for Your Life*, O. Carl Simonton's *Getting Well Again*, and books by psychiatrist Karl Menninger. You will also do well to read the works of doctors Larry Dossey, Andrew Weil, Deepak Chopra, and many others. Again, all you need to do is go to the bookstore and look for the subject you want to learn about—whether it's herbal medicine, acupuncture, holistic medicine, or any other type of alternative therapy. Call the organizations that support people with the specific problem you want help with and ask them what books and tapes are available. Be sure to speak with the natives and ask for their recommendations. Find out about people who have survived a loss or illness, such as Lance Armstrong, the champion cyclist. Read their books and see what helped them.

Some of the magazines I find most helpful are: *Advances in Mind-Body Medicine, Alternative Therapies in Health and Medicine, Science & Spirit, Spirituality & Health, Discover,* and *Psychology Today.*

The International Society for the Study of Subtle Energies and Energy Medicine (ISSSEEM) and the American Holistic Medical Association (AHMA) are good resources that can expand your horizons. Keep in touch with the National Center for Complementary and Alternative Medicine, a component of the National Institutes of Health, and their research (Website: **www.nccam.nih.gov**).

A program called "Touch for Life" provides a kit that will show you how to create positive, therapeutic, nonthreatening sensory experiences in health and attitude for all ages—from infants to seniors. Information about this and other programs can be found on the Kisses from Heaven Website (**www.kissesfromheaven.com**).

You can use the Internet to gather more information and learn about your treatment options—but be careful. Everywhere you search, whether on the Web or in a library, there will be some closed-minded people on both sides of the healing fence. If someone guarantees you a certain result, be wary. Some of the people in chat rooms don't have the illness they claim to have, and some may depress instead of help you. Remember: You're looking for your *own* path.

Finally—don't laugh—I consider the ultimate resources to be newspapers such as *The New York Times* and *USA Today*. As I'm writing this, *USA Today* is reporting on a study of surgery patients who used guided-imagery tapes. Sound familiar? The study found that patients who used visualization tapes healed faster and had less pain than the control group. Many other studies substantiate the benefits and healing approaches we've written about—from group support to the effect of attitude on healing and survival—and you can read about them in the paper.

You now have the information you need to organize your own healing. Now go do it—then perhaps you'll be able to write your own book about how to heal.

❦

Yosaif's Resource List

Here are some resources I recommend:

Bedscapes®
146 Spencer Road
Glenford, NY 12433
info@bedscapes.com
(e-mail)
www.bedscapes.com

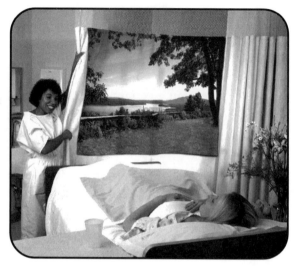

Choice Magazine Listening
(This service offers free magazine readings on tape for people who are blind,
visually impaired, or physically disabled.)
85 Channel Drive
Port Washington, NY 11050
516-883-8280 or 888-724-6423 (phone)
516-944-6849 (fax)
choicemag@aol.com (e-mail)
www.choicemagazinelistening.org

National Family Caregivers Association
10400 Connecticut Avenue, #500
Kensington, MD 20895-3944
800-896-3650 (phone)
301-942-2302 (fax)
info@nfcacares.org (e-mail)
www.nfcacares.org

Family Caregiver Alliance
690 Market St., Ste. 600
San Francisco, CA 94104
415-434-3388 (phone)
415-435-3308 (fax)
info@caregiver.org (e-mail)
www.caregiver.org

National Stroke Association
9707 E. Easter Lane
Englewood, Co. 80112
800-STROKES or 303-649-9299 (phone)
303-649-1328 (fax)
www.stroke.org

Re: Pain Management
National Pain Foundation
www.painconnection.org
866-590-PAIN (7246)

American Pain Foundation
www.painfoundation.org
888-615-PAIN (7246)

Managing Pain Before It Manages You,
Margaret Caudill, M.D., Ph.D. (Guilford Press, 2001)

The War on Pain, Scott Fishman, M.D., with Lisa Berger
(Quill, 2001)

You Don't Have to Hurt, Peter Staats, M.D., with Philip Bashe (Workman
Publishing, available in 2004)

Re: Cancer—Pioneering Grassroots Advocacy
1 in 9: The Long Island Breast Cancer Action Coalition
www.1in9.org

Hewlett House Cancer Resource Center
www.hewletthouse.org

Re: Informed Decision Making
Health Commons Institute
135 Marginal Way #375
P.O. Box 9715
Portland, ME 04104-5015
207-772-1354 (phone)
207-772-1355 (fax)
www.healthcommons.org

Re: Humanizing Health Care
The Caritas Project
www.thecaritasproject.info

Re: Long-Term Care
The Eden Alternative
www.edenalt.com

Re: Healing Arts
Society for the Arts in Healthcare
www.societyartshealthcare.org

Art Folks
www.artfolks.com

ENTITLEMENT LEARNER'S PERMIT

This is to certify that _____was born a totally and unconditionally lovable human being. Being aware of the imperfections humans may manifest, we nevertheless declare for all to acknowledge that _____is entitled to be embraced with love, to be treated with respect and dignity, and to never have to apologize for asking for what he or she needs.

This permit is valid until the aforementioned wakes up to the fact that such entitlement is his or her birthright.

_____

Bernie Siegel, M.D.,
Doctor of Unconditional Love

_____

Yosaif August,
Commissioner of Birthrights

AFTERWORD

Passwords

We considered closing with a regular afterword or epilogue, but those didn't seem quite right for a book about embarking on a healing journey. You see, when you travel outside your homeland, you need a passport. We decided that you might not need a pass*port* on this trip, but you could probably benefit from having some pass*words* to help you enter new territories. The passwords here should help guide you when you're feeling tested by the new landscape.

Your first password is *training*. Taking a healing journey is like being in training, and reading about healing is only a starting point. You'll need supportive coaching, good technique, a lot of practice, and the willingness to say yes to your inner self. We've done our best here to empower you with information and techniques, and as you continue your training, you may reach a point when you'll be teaching others by your example. If you enjoy being a teacher, then feel free to share what you've learned— but don't try to convince others that what heals you will heal them. Each of us must make his or her own way in this new land we're entering.

You may encounter guides who can teach you, but you still have to find your *intuition*. If you were participating in a dogsled race across Alaska, you'd want a well-trained lead dog who has inner wisdom about which path to take. That wise sled dog already exists—within your heart. Follow your instincts when you have to make decisions about what's right for you, and you'll never take the wrong path to healing.

You'll also need a *vision* in order to act on the facts you gather. Intelligent people are quick to apprehend new information, but we want you to be more than intelligent—we want you to be wise. Those who are wise set goals and envision what it will take to reach them.

We hope that our information will give you a glimpse of what it's like to have a healed life, but know that your vision won't become a reality unless you *work* on it. It's not enough to read or research, you need to take action. On the other hand, work without vision is drudgery. To find a healing path and stay on it, you need to combine the two.

So your passwords for your healing journey are *training, intuition, vision*, and *work*. Keep those passwords in mind, along with a few others that need no explanation: *love, laughter,* and *miracles*. And please accept our blessings for your journey.

— **Bernie & Yosaif**

SELF-HELP RESOURCES

The following list of resources can be used to access information on a variety of issues. The addresses and telephone numbers listed are for the national headquarters; look in your local yellow pages under "Community Services" for resources closer to your area.

In addition to the following groups, other self-help organizations may be available in your area to assist your healing and recovery for a particular life crisis not listed here. Consult your telephone directory, call a counseling center or help line near you, or contact:

AIDS

(United States)

CDC National AIDS Hotline
(800) 342-2437

Caring for Babies with AIDS
P.O. Box 35135
Los Angeles, CA 90035
(323) 931-9828
www.caring4babieswithaids.org

Children with AIDS (CWA)
Project of America
P.O. Box 23778
Tempe, AZ 85285
(800) 866-AIDS (24-hour hotline)
www.aidskids.org

Elizabeth Glaser Pediatric AIDS
Foundation
2950 31st St., #125
Santa Monica, CA 90405
(888) 499-HOPE (4673)
www.pedaids.org

**The Names Project Foundation—
AIDS Memorial Quilt**
P.O. Box 5552
Atlanta, GA 31107
(800) 872-6263
www.aidsquilt.org

Project Inform
205 13th St., Ste. 2001
San Francisco, CA 94103
(800) 822-7422 (treatment hotline)
(415) 558-9051 (S.F. and Intl.)
www.projectinform.org

Spanish HIV/STD/AIDS Hotline
(800) 344-7432

**TTY (Hearing Impaired)
AIDS Hotline
(CDC National HIV/AIDS)**
(800) 243-7889

(United Kingdom)

National AIDS Helpline
0 800 567123
www.healthwise.org.uk

National AIDS Trust
New City Cloisters
196 Old Street
London EC1V 9F4
020 7814 6767
www.nat.org.uk

(Canada)

Canadian AIDS Society
4th Floor—309 rue Cooper Street
Ottawa ON K2P 0G5
(613)230-3580

Health Canada
HIV/AIDS
www.aidsida.com

ALCOHOL ABUSE

(United States)

**Al-Anon Family Group
Headquarters**
1600 Corporate Landing Parkway
Virginia Beach, VA 23454-5617
(888) 4AL-ANON
www.al-anon.alateen.org

Alcoholics Anonymous (AA)
General Service Office
475 Riverside Dr., 11th Floor
New York, NY 10115
(212) 870-3400
www.alcoholics-anonymous.org

Children of Alcoholics Foundation
164 W. 74th St.
New York, NY 10023
(800) 359-COAF
www.coaf.org

**Mothers Against Drunk Driving
(MADD)**
P.O. Box 541688
Dallas, TX 75354
(800) GET-MADD (438-6233)
www.madd.org

**National Association of Children
of Alcoholics (NACoA)**
11426 Rockville Pike, #100
Rockville, MD 20852
(301) 468-0985
(888) 554-2627
www.nacoa.net

**National Clearinghouse for
Alcohol and Drug Information
(NCADI)**
P.O. Box 2345
Rockville, MD 20847
(800) 729-6686
www.health.org

**National Council on Alcoholism
and Drug Dependence (NCADD)**
20 Exchange Pl., Ste. 2902
New York, NY 10005
(212) 269-7797
(800) NCA-CALL (24-hour hotline)
www.ncadd.org

Women for Sobriety
P.O. Box 618
Quakertown, PA 18951
(215) 536-8026
www.womenforsobriety.org

(United Kingdom)

Alcohol Concern
020 7922 8667
www.alcoholconcern.org.uk

Alcoholics Anonymous
General Service Office
P.O. Box 1, Stonebow House
Stonebow YO1 7NJ
(44) 01904-644026
www.alcoholics-anonymous.org.uk

Healthwise Drinkline
0800 917 8282
www.healthwise.org.uk

(Canada)

Alcoholics Anonymous
www.aa.org/index.html

Al-Anon/Alateen
(800) 714-7498
(for information and materials)
(800) 443-4525
(for meeting locations)

**Canadian Center on Substance
Abuse**
75 Albert Street, Ste. 300
Ottawa ON K1P 5E7
(613) 235-4048
www.ccsa.ca

**Canadians for Safe and
Sober Driving**
P.O. Box 397
Station "A"
Brampton ON L6V 2L3
(905) 793-4233
www.add.ca

ALZHEIMER'S DISEASE

(United States)

Alzheimer's Association
919 N. Michigan Ave., Ste. 1100
Chicago, IL 60611
(800) 272-3900
www.alz.org

**Alzheimer's Disease Education
and Referral Center**
P.O. Box 8250
Silver Spring, MD 20907
(800) 438-4380
adear@alzheimers.org

Eldercare Locator
330 Independence Ave., SW
Washington, DC 20201
(800) 677-1116
www.eldercare.gov

(United Kingdom)

Alzheimer's Society
Gordon House
10 Greencoat Place
London SW1P 1PH
020 7606 0606
www.alzheimers.org.uk

(Canada)

Alzeheimer Society of Canada
20 Eglinton Avenue W., Suite 1200
Toronto ON M4R 1K8
(800) 616-8816
www.alzheimer.ca

CANCER

(Unites States)

Candlelighters
Childhood Cancer Foundation
CCCF National Office
P.O. Box 498
Kensington, MD 20895-0498
(800) 366-2223
(301) 962-3521 (fax)
www.candlelighters.org

National Cancer Institute
(800) 4-CANCER
www.nci.nih.gov

(United Kingdom)

CancerHelp UK
Institute for Cancer Studies
University of Birmingham
Edgbaston
Birmingham B15 2TA
www.cancerhelp.org.uk

(Canada)

Canadian Cancer Society
(888) 939-3333
www.cancer.ca

CHILDREN'S ISSUES

Child Molestation

(United States)

Childhelp USA/Child Abuse Hotline
15757 N. 78th St.
Scottsdale, AZ 85260
(800) 422-4453
www.childhelpusa.org

Prevent Child Abuse America
200 South Michigan Ave.,
17th Floor
Chicago, IL 60604
(312) 663-3520
www.preventchildabuse.org

(United Kingdom)

Childline
Royal Mail Building, 2nd Floor
Studd Street
London N1 OQW
0800 1111 (helpline)
0800 400 222 (text phone service)
www.childline.org.uk

National Society for the Prevention of Cruelty to Children (NSPCC)
Weston House
42 Curtains Road
London EC2A 3NH
020 7825 2500 (administration)
0808 800 5000 (helpline)

(Canada)

Child Abuse Hotline
(800) 387-5437

Kids Help Phone
(800) 668-6868
http://kidshelp.simaptico.ca

**The Canadian Society for the
Prevention of Cruelty to Children**
Box 700, 356 First Street
Midland ON L4R 4P4
(705)526-5647

Crisis Intervention

(United States)

**Girls and Boys Town National
Hotline**
(800) 448-3000
www.boystown.org

Children of the Night
14530 Sylvan St.
Van Nuys, CA 91411
(800) 551-1300
www.childrenofthenight.org

Covenant House Hotline
(800) 999-9999
www.covenanthouse.org

Kid Save Line
(800) 543-7283
www.kidspeace.org

Youth Nineline
(referrals for parents/teens about
drugs, homelessness, runaways)
(800) 999-9999

(United Kingdom)

Barnardo's
Tanner's Lane
Barkingside
Ilford IG6 1QG
020 8550 8822
www.barnardos.org.uk

Childline
Royal Mail Building, 2nd Floor
Studd Street
London N1 OQW
0800 1111 (helpline)
0800 400 222 (text phone service)
www.childline.org.uk

The Prince's Trust
18 Park Square East
London NW1 4LH
020 7543 1234
www.princes-trust.org.uk

Safe in the City
020 7922 5710
www.safeinthecity.org.uk

(Canada)

Covenant House
575 Drake Street
Vancouver BC V6B 4K8
(604) 685-7474
www.covenenthousebc.org

Covenant House
20 Gerrard Street East
Toronto, ON M5B 2P3
(416) 598-4898
www.covenanthouse.org

Kids Help Phone
(800) 668-6868
http://kidshelp.simpatico.ca

Missing Children

(United States)

Missing Children . . .
HELP Center
410 Ware Blvd., Ste. 710
Tampa, FL 33619
(800) USA-KIDS
www.800usakids.org

National Center for Missing &
Exploited Children
699 Prince St.
Alexandria, VA 22314
(800) 843-5678 (24-hour hotline)
www.missingkids.org

(United Kingdom)

National Missing Persons Helpline
0500 700 700
www.missingpersons.org

UK Missing and Exploited
Children
http://uk.missingkids.com

(Canada)

Child Find Canada
1-1808 Main Street
Winnipeg MB R2V 2A3
(204) 339-5584
www.childfind.ca

Missing Children
Society of Canada
Suite 219, 3501 - 23 Street NE
Calgary AB T2E 6V8

(800) 661-6160
www.mcsc.ca

Children with Serious Illnesses
(fulfilling wishes):

(United States)

Brass Ring Society
National Headquarters
551 E. Semoran Blvd., Ste. E-5
Fern Park, FL 32730
(407) 339-6188
(800) 666-WISH
www.worldramp.net/brassring

Make-a-Wish Foundation
3550 N. Central Ave., Ste. 300
Phoenix, AZ 85012
(800) 722-WISH (9474)
www.wish.org

(United Kingdom)

Make-a-Wish Foundation UK
01276 24127
www.make-a-wish.org.uk

Starlight Foundation
11-15 Emerald Street
London WC1N 3QL
020 7430 1642
www.starlight.org.uk

(Canada)

Make-a-Wish Foundation of
Canada
2239 Oak Street
Vancouver BC V6H 3W6
(888) 822-9474
www.makeawish.ca

CO-DEPENDENCY

Co-Dependents Anonymous
P.O. Box 33577
Phoenix, AZ 85067
(602) 277-7991
www.codependents.org

Co-Dependents Anonymous World Service, Inc.
P.O. Box 7051
Thomaston, GA USA 30286-0025
(706) 648-6868
www.wscoda.org

DEATH/GRIEVING/SUICIDE

(United States)

AARP Grief and Loss Programs
(202) 434-2260
(800) 424-3410
www.aarp.org/griefandloss

Grief Recovery Institute
P.O. Box 6061-382
Sherman Oaks, CA 91413
(818) 907-9600
www/grief-recovery.com

National Hospice and Palliative Care Organization
1700 Diagonal Rd., Ste. 300
Alexandria, VA 22314
(703) 837-1500
www.nhpco.org

Parents of Murdered Children
(recovering from violent death of friend or family member)
100 E 8th St., Ste. B41

Cincinnati, OH 45202
(513) 721-5683
(888) 818-POMC
www.pomc.com

SIDS (Sudden Infant Death Syndrome) Alliance
1314 Bedford Ave., Ste. 210
Baltimore, MD 21208
(800) 221-7437
www.sidsalliance.org

Suicide Awareness Voices of Education (SAVE)
Minneapolis, MN 55424
(952) 946-7998

Suicide National Hotline
(800) 784-2433

(United Kingdom)

The Compassionate Friends
53 North Street
Bristol BS3 1EN
0117 953 9639 (helpline)
0177 966 5202 (administration)
www.compassionatefriends.org.uk

Winston's Wish
The Clara Burgess Centre
Gloucestershire Royal Hospital
Great Western Road
Gloucester GL1 3NN
+44 (0) 1452 394377 (general inquiries)
0845 20 30 40 5 (family line)
www.winstonswish.org.uk

(Canada)

**Canadian Hospice Palliative
Care Association**
43 Bruyère St., Ste. 131 C
Ottawa, ON K1N 5C8
(800) 668-2785
www.cpa.net

**Seasons Centre for
Grieving Children**
4 Alliance Boulevard, Unit 7
Barrie ON L4M 5J1
(705) 721-5437
www.seasonscentre.com

**Suicide Information and
Education Centre**
#201 1615-10th Avenue SW
Calgary AB T3C 0J7
www.suicideinfo.ca

DEBTS

(United States)

**Consumer Credit
Counseling Service
Credit Referral**
(800) 388-CCCS

Debtors Anonymous
General Service Office
P.O. Box 920888
Needham, MA 02492-0009
(781) 453-2743
www.debtorsanonymous.org

DIABETES

(United States)

American Diabetes Association
(800) 342-2383
www.diabetes.org

(United Kingdom)

Diabetes UK
10 Parkway
London NW1 7AA
020 7424 1000
www.diabetesuk.org

(Canada)

Canadian Diabetes Association
(800) 226-8464
www.diabetes.ca

DOMESTIC VIOLENCE

(United States)

**National Coalition Against
Domestic Violence**
P.O. Box 18749
Denver, CO 80218
(303) 831-9251
www.ncadv.org

**National Domestic Violence
Hotline**
P.O. Box 161810
Austin, TX 78716
(800) 799-SAFE (24-hour hotline)
(800) 787-3224 (TTY)
www.ndvh.org

(United Kingdom)

Women's Aid
P.O. Box 391
Bristol BS99 7WS
08457 023 468 (helpline)
0117 944 441 (administration)
www.womensaid.org.uk

Victim Support
0845 30 30 900 (helpline)

(Canada)

Evolve (KLINIC)
870 Portage Ave.
Winnipeg, MB MR3G 0P1
(204) 784-4090
www.klinic.mb.ca

**National Domestic
Violence Hotline**
(800) 363-9010

Safe Home
(888) 926-0301

DRUG ABUSE

(United States)

**Cocaine Anonymous National
Referral Line**
(800) 347-8998

**National Helpline of Phoenix
House**
(cocaine abuse hotline)
(800) 262-2463
(800) COCAINE
www.drughelp.org

**National Institute of Drug Abuse
(NIDA)**
6001 Executive Blvd., Rm. 5213
Bethesda, MD 20892-9561
Parklawn Building
(301) 443-6245 (for information)
(800) 662-4357 (for help)
www.nida.nih.gov

World Service Office, Inc.
3740 Overland Ave., Ste. C
Los Angeles, CA 90034-6337
(310) 559-5833

(United Kingdom)

National Drug Helpline
0800 77 66 00
www.ndhl.org.uk

**The Centre for Recovery
Cyswllt Ceredigion Contact**
49 North Parade
Ceredigion SY23 2JN
01970 626470
www.recovery.org.uk

**Narcotics Anonymous—
UK Region**
020 7730 0009
www.ukna.org

(Canada)

**Canadian Assembly Narcotics
Anonymous**
CANA/ACNA
P.O. Box 25073 RPO West Kildonan
Winnipeg MB R2V 4C7
www.cana-acna.org

Canadian Centre on Substance Abuse
75 Albert St., Ste. 300
Ottawa ON K1P 5E7
(613) 235-4048
www.ccsa.ca

EATING DISORDERS

(United States)

Overeaters Anonymous
National Office
P.O. Box 44020
Rio Rancho, NM 87174-4020
(505) 891-2664
www.overeatersanonymous.org

(United Kingdom)

Eating Disorders Association
103 Prince of Wales Road
Norwich NR1 1DW
0845 634 1414 (adults)
0845 634 7650 (youth)
www.edauk.com

(Canada)

National Eating Disorder Information Center
CW 1- 211 Elizabeth Street
Toronto, ON M5G 2C4
(866) 633-4240
www.nedic.ca

GAMBLING

Gamblers Anonymous
International Service Office
P.O. Box 17173
Los Angeles, CA 90017
(213) 386-8789
www.gamblersanonymous.org

Gamblers Anonymous UK
P.O. Box 88
London SW10 0EU
08700 50 88 80
www.gamblersanonymous.org.uk

Gamblers Anonymous Canada
(by Province)
www.gamlersanonymous.org.mtgdir
CAN.html

HEALTH ISSUES

(United States)

American Chronic Pain Association
P.O. Box 850
Rocklin, CA 95677
(916) 632-0922
www.theacpa.org

American Holistic Health Association
P.O. Box 17400
Anaheim, CA 92817
(714) 779-6152
www.ahha.org

The Chopra Center at La Costa Resort and Spa
Deepak Chopra, M.D.

7321 Estrella Del Mar
Carlsbad, CA 92009
(760) 931-7524
www.chopra.com

Hippocrates Health Institute
(A favorite annual retreat
for Louise Hay)
1443 Palmdale Court
West Palm Beach, FL 33411
(800) 842-2125
www.hippocratesinst.com

Hospicelink
190 W. Brook Rd.
Essex, CT 06426
(800) 331-1620

Institute for Noetic Sciences
101 San Antonio Rd.
Petaluma, CA 94952
(707) 775-3500
www.noetic.org

The Mind-Body Medical Institute
110 Francis St., Ste. 1A
Boston, MA 02215
(617) 632-9530 (press 1)
www.mbmi.org

**National Health Information
Center**
P.O. Box 1133
Washington, DC 20013-1133
(800) 336-4797
www.health.gov/NHIC

Optimum Health Institute
(Louise Hay loves this place!)
6970 Central Ave.
Lemon Grove, CA 91945
(619) 464-3346
www.optimumhealth.org

**Preventive Medicine
Research Institute**
Dean Ornish, M.D.
900 Bridgeway, Ste. 2
Sausalito, CA 94965
(415) 332-2525
www.pmri.org

(United Kingdom)

**National Health Service
(NHS) Direct**
0845 4647 (24-hour nurse
advice line)
www.nhsdirect.nhs.uk

UK Health Centre
www.healthcentre.org.uk

(Canada)

Health Canada
Minister's Office
Brooke Claxton Bldg.,
Tunney's Pasture
PL 0906C
Ottawa, ON K1A 0K9
(613) 952-1154 (fax)
www.hc-sc.gc.ca

HOUSING RESOURCES

(United States)

Acorn
(nonprofit network of low-
and moderate-income housing)
739 8th St., S.E.
Washington, DC 20003
(202) 547-9292

(United Kingdom)

The Abbeyfield Society
(for elderly people)
The Abbeyfield House
53 Victoria St.
St Albans
Herts AL1 3UW
01727 857536
www.abbeyfield.com

Centrepoint (for young people)
Neil House
7 Whitechapel Road
London E1 1DU
020 7426 5300
www.centrepoint.org.uk

Shelterline
0808 8000 4444
www.shelter.org.uk

(Canada)

**Abbeyfield Houses
Society of Canada**
Box 1, 427 Bloor St. West
Toronto, ON M5S 1X7
(416) 920-7483
www.abbeyfield.ca

**Canada Mortgage and
Housing Corporation**
700 Montreal Rd.
Ottawa, ON K1A 0P7
(613) 748-2000
www.cmhc-schl.gc.ca

IMPOTENCE

(United States)

Impotence Institute of America
8201 Corporate Dr., Ste. 320
Landover, MD 20715
(800) 669-1603
www.impotenceworld.org

(United Kingdom)

The Impotence Association
P.O. Box 10296
London SW17 9WH
020 8767 7791
www.impotence.org.uk

MENTAL HEALTH

(United States)

**American Psychiatric Association
of America**
1400 "K" St. NW
Washington, DC 20005
(888) 357-7924
www.psych.org

**Anxiety Disorders Association
of America**
11900 Parklawn Dr., Ste. 100
Rockville, MD 20852
(301) 231-9350
www.adaa.org

**The Help Center of the American
Psychological Association**
(800) 964-2000
www.helping.apa.org

The International Society for Mental Health Online
www.ismho.org

Knowledge Exchange Network
www.mentalhealth.org

National Center for Post-Traumatic Stress Disorder (PTSD)
(802) 296-5132
www.ncptsd.org

National Alliance for the Mentally Ill
2107 Wilson Blvd., Ste. 300
Arlington, VA 22201
(800) 950-6264
www.nami.org

National Depressive and Manic-Depressive Association
730 N. Franklin St., Ste. 501
Chicago, IL 60610
(800) 826-3632
www.ndmda.org

National Institute of Mental Health
6001 Executive Blvd.
Room 8184, MSC 9663
Bethesda, MD 20892
(301) 443-4513
(301) 443-8431 (TTY)
www.nimh.nih.gov

(United Kingdom)

Mind (The National Association for Mental Health)
15-19 Broadway
London E15 4BQ
020 8519 2122
www.mind.org.uk

Sane
1st Floor
Cityside House
40 Adler Street
London E1 1EE
020 7375 1002
0845 767 8000
(saneline— open noon–2 A.M.)
www.sane.org.uk

(Canada)

Canadian Mental Health Association
2160 Yonge Street, 3rd Floor
Toronto, ON M4S 2Z3
(416) 484-7750
www.cmha.ca

Mood Disorders Association of Canada
4-1000 Notre Dame Ave.
Winnipeg, MB R3E 0N3
(800) 263-1460

PET BEREAVEMENT

(United States)

Bide-A-Wee Foundation
410 E. 38th St.
New York, NY 10016
(212) 532-6395

Grief Recovery Hotline
(800) 445-4808

Holistic Animal Consulting Centre
29 Lyman Ave.
Staten Island, NY 10305
(718) 720-5548

(United Kingdom)

Animal Samaritans
52 Verdant Lane
London SE3 1LF
020 8852 9132
www.animalsamaritans.org.uk

(Canada)

Pet Therapy Society of Northern Alberta
330, 9768 170 Street
Edmonton, AB T5T L54
(780) 413-4682
http://paws.shopalberta.com/
PTRemember.htm

RAPE/SEXUAL ISSUES

(United States)

Rape, Abuse, and Incest National Network
(800) 656-4673
www.rainn.org

SafePlace
P.O. Box 19454
Austin, TX 78760
(512) 440-7273

National Council on Sexual Addictions and Compulsivity
P.O. Box 725544
Atlanta, GA 31139
(770) 541-9912
www.ncsac.org

Sexually Transmitted Disease Referral
(800) 227-8922

(United Kingdom)

Rape Crisis Federation of Wales and England
7 Mansfield Rd.
Nottingham NG1 3FB
0115 934 8474
www.rapecrisis.co.uk

Rape and Sexual Abuse Counseling
01962 848018 (administration)
01962 848024 (helpline for women)
01962 848027 (helpline for men)
http://rasc.org.uk

(Canada)

Canadian Association of Sexual Assault Centres
77 East 20th Ave.
Vancouver BC V5V 1L7
(604) 876-2622
www.casac.ca

Let's Protect
(list of resources for women in Canada and the U.S.)
www.letsprotect.com

SMOKING

(United States)

Nicotine Anonymous World Services
419 Main St., PMB #370
Huntington Beach, CA 92648
(415) 750-0328
www.nicotine-anonymous.org

(United Kingdom)

Quit
0800 00 22 00
www.quit.org.uk

(Canada)

Lung Association
3 Raymond St., Ste. 300
Ottawa ON KR1 1A3
(613) 569-6411
www.lung.ca/smoking

STRESS REDUCTION

(United States)

**The Biofeedback &
Psychophysiology Clinic**
The Menninger Clinic
P.O. Box 829
Topeka, KS 66601-0829
(800) 351-9058
www.menninger.edu

New York Open Center
(In-depth workshops to
invigorate the spirit)
83 Spring St.
New York, NY 10012
(212) 219-2527
www.opencenter.org

Omega Institute
(a healing, spiritual retreat
community)
150 Lake Dr.
Rhinebeck, NY 12572-3212
(845) 266-4444 (info)
(800) 944-1001 (to enroll)
www.eomega.org

The Stress Reduction Clinic
Center for Mindfulness
University of Massachusetts
Medical Center
55 Lake Ave. North
Worcester, MA 01655
(508) 856-2656

(United Kingdom)

**International Stress Management
Association**
P.O. Box 348
Waltham Cross EN8 8ZL
07000 780430
www.isma.org.uk

TEEN HELP

**ADOL: Adolescent Directory
Online**
Includes information on eating disorders, depression, and teen pregnancy.
www.education.indiana.edu/cas/adol/
adol.html

Al-Anon/Alateen
1600 Corporate Landing Parkway
Virginia Beach, VA 23454-5617
(888) 425-2666
(888) 4AL-ANON
www.al-anon.alateen.org

**Focus Adolescent Services: Eating
Disorders**
(877) 362-8727
www.focusas.com/EatingDisorders.html

Future Point
A nonprofit organization that offers
message boards and chat rooms to
empower teens in the academic
world and beyond.
www.futurepoint.org

Kids in Trouble Help Page
Child abuse, depression, suicide, and runaway resources, with links and hotline numbers.
www.geocities.com/EnchantedForest/2910

Planned Parenthood
810 Seventh Ave.
New York, NY 10019
(212) 541-7800
(800) 230-PLAN
www.plannedparenthood.org

SafeTeens.com
Provides lessons on online safety and privacy; also has resources for homework and fun on the Web.
www.safeteens.com

TeenCentral.net
This site is written by and about teens.
Includes celebrity stories, real-teen tales, an anonymous help-line, and crisis counseling.
www.teencentral.net

TeenOutReach.com
Includes all kinds of information geared at teens, from sports to entertainment to help with drugs and eating disorders.
www.teenoutreach.com

Hotlines for Teenagers

(United States)

Girls and Boys Town National Hotline
(800) 448-3000

Childhelp National Child Abuse Hotline/ Voices for Children
(800) 422-4453
(800) 4ACHILD

Just for Kids Hotline
(888) 594-5437
(888) 594-KIDS

National Child Abuse Hotline
(800) 792-5200

National Runaway Hotline
(800) 621-4000

National Youth Crisis Hotline
(800) 448-4663
(800) HIT HOME

Suicide Prevention Hotline
(800) 827-7571

(United Kingdom)

Alateen (for teens with alcohol concerns)
020 7403 0888

Anti Bullying Campaign
(counseling and advice)
020 7378 1446

Careline (counseling and advice)
020 8514 1177

Family-line UK (for families in crisis)
0845 756 7800

National Association for Children of Alcoholics
0800 567123

(Canada)

**AIDS/ Sexually Transmitted
Diseases Info**
(800) 772-2437

Gambling Help Line
(800) 665-9676

Kid's Help Phone
(800) 668-6868

ABOUT THE AUTHORS

Bernie Siegel, M.D., is a retired general/pediatric surgeon who is now involved in humanizing medical care and medical education. In 1978, he originated Exceptional Cancer Patients (ECaP), a specific form of individual and group therapy. He is the author of *Love, Medicine & Miracles; Peace, Love & Healing; How to Live Between Office Visits;* and *Prescriptions for Living.* Bernie and his wife, Bobbie, live in Connecticut and have five children and eight grandchildren. Bernie embraces a philosophy of living and dying that stands at the forefront of the ethical and spiritual issues our society and medical care grapple with today. Website: **www.ecap-online.org**

Yosaif August is a "bedside environmentalist," promoting the importance of improving the bedside experiences of patients. In 1995, because of his own experiences as a hospitalized patient and caregiver for his parents, he left his corporate consulting business to become a full-time health advocate and social entrepreneur. He is the president of Healing Environments, International, and the inventor of Bedscapes®, which helps patients by turning the conventional cubicle curtain into a healing-friendly space. Yosaif has two grown children and a grandson and lives in Woodstock, New York, with his wife, Tsurah, and two cats. Website: **www.bedscapes.com**

HAY HOUSE TITLES OF RELATED INTEREST

Books

Deep Healing, by Emmett E. Miller, M.D.

Doctors Cry, Too: *Essays from the Heart of a Physician,*
by Frank H. Boehm, M.D.

Heal Your Body, by Louise L. Hay

The Power of Touch: *The Basis for Survival, Health, Intimacy,
and Emotional Well-Being,* by Phyllis K. Davis, Ph.D.

The Power of the Mind to Heal:
Renewing Body, Mind, and Spirit,
by Joan Borysenko, Ph.D., and Miroslav Borysenko, Ph.D.

The Wellness Book, by John Randolph Price

Card Decks

Healing Cards: *A Daily Practice for
Maintaining Spiritual Balance,*
by Caroline Myss and Peter Occhiogrosso

Healing the Mind and Spirit Cards, by Brian L. Weiss, M.D.

Healthy Body Cards, by Louise L. Hay

I Can Do It® Cards: *Affirmations for Health,* by Louise L. Hay

Miracle Cards, by Marianne Williamson

All of the above are available at your local bookstore,
or may be ordered through Hay House, Inc. (see info on last page).

❧

We hope you enjoyed this Hay House book.
If you would like to receive a free catalog featuring
additional Hay House books and products, or
if you would like information about the
Hay Foundation, please contact:

Hay House, Inc.
P.O. Box 5100
Carlsbad, CA 92018-5100

(760) 431-7695 or (800) 654-5126
(760) 431-6948 (fax) or (800) 650-5115 (fax)
www.hayhouse.com

❧

Published and distributed in Australia by:
Hay House Australia, Ltd., 18/36 Ralph St., Alexandria NSW 2015
Phone: 612-9669-4299 • *Fax:* 612-9669-4144
www.hayhouse.com.au

Published and Distributed in the United Kingdom by:
Hay House UK, Ltd. • Unit 202, Canalot Studios
222 Kensal Rd., London W10 5BN • *Phone:* 44-20-8962-1230
Fax: 44-20-8962-1239 • www.hayhouse.co.uk

Distributed in Canada by: Raincoast
9050 Shaughnessy St., Vancouver, B.C. V6P 6E5
Phone: (604) 323-7100 • *Fax:* (604) 323-2600

❧

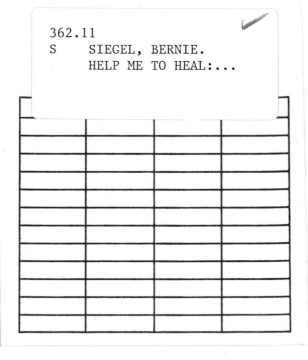